Public Health, Humanities and Magical Realism

This book calls for a reconceptualisation of the public health evidence base to include crucial forms of creative and relational data about people's lived and felt experiences that cannot be accessed through the biomedical approach to generating and using evidence.

Drawing from the author's ethical, ontological, and epistemological dilemmas when studying controversial topics and methodological evaluation framework to measure impacts of creative community engagement, the book argues that traditional methodologies and conceptualisations of evidence have the potential to exacerbate health inequalities by excluding and misrepresenting minorities. Fantastical realities based on "truthful" research findings are intertwined with traditional public health approaches through artistic engagement with so-called hard-to-reach groups. Working with their (sur)real life stories, the author reflects on how the population's breadth is inadequately reflected, which threatens validity and generalisability in public health research and decision-making.

Through different ways of knowing (epistemology) and different ways of being (ontology), this book shows how to design studies, make recommendations, and adapt services that are aligned with views and experiences of those living on the margins and beyond. As such, it is an essential read for public health researchers and students.

Marisa de Andrade is an academic in health policy at the University of Edinburgh. She is Programme Director for the MSc by Research in Health Humanities and Arts, Programme Director for the PhD in Health in Social Science, Associate Director for the Centre for Creative-Relational Inquiry, and Co-director at the Binks Hub, working with communities to co-produce a programme of research and knowledge exchange that promotes social justice, relational research methods, and human flourishing. Marisa has led several traditional and community-based, arts-informed public health studies. She is currently PI on an Arts and Humanities Research Council (AHRC) collaborative place-based grant putting the arts at the helm of strategic decision-making across multiple sectors, including health and social care, employability, education, and social justice.

Routledge Studies in Public Health

Public Health, Humanities and Magical Realism

A Creative-Relational Approach to
Researching Human Experience

Marisa de Andrade

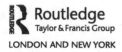
Routledge
Taylor & Francis Group

LONDON AND NEW YORK

First published 2023
by Routledge
4 Park Square, Milton Park, Abingdon, Oxon OX14 4RN

and by Routledge
605 Third Avenue, New York, NY 10158

Routledge is an imprint of the Taylor & Francis Group, an informa business

© 2023 Marisa de Andrade

British Library Cataloguing-in-Publication Data
A catalogue record for this book is available from the British Library

Library of Congress Cataloging-in-Publication Data
A catalog record for this book has been requested

ISBN: 978-1-032-05189-5 (hbk)
ISBN: 978-1-032-05190-1 (pbk)
ISBN: 978-1-003-19648-8 (ebk)

DOI: 10.4324/9781003196488

Typeset in Goudy
by Apex CoVantage, LLC

To the system, and the humans who believe in the magic, kindness, and power in every relationship within it

Contents

Acknowledgements

Time moves forward, it never moves back

To Rocco, my love, my greatest teacher, mum, dad, family, friends, nearest – including those who are far – and dearest. Thank you to the person at my graduation who told me, and thousands of others, to *"be bold – you never know when you're walking through an open door"*. I've held that thought in my mind as I've stumbled into research and personal dilemmas, as I've tried to make sense of internal and external realities, as I've allowed myself to integrate different disciplines and parts of myself into methodology and into life. Thanks to the funders – the individuals – who believed in something I couldn't fully articulate at the time. Off the top of my head, from NHS Greater Glasgow and Clyde back in the day, Fiona, Rebecca, Ruth, Lara, Heather, Paul. Keith from social work for being there and opening doors despite being so, so busy. From The Conservation Volunteers, Dom and the team, especially the person who inspired the pine martin trial by simply telling their truth. From Bethany Christian Trust, Shirley, who led me to Paul, who led me to his incredible team – Colin, Felicity, Jean, Rilza and others over the years. Sean Kerwin, "the Measuring Humanity producer", who continues to listen as I riff academic speak and helps me turn it into decipherable, artistic visual and audio sound bites. To Belle Jones, Audrey Tait and Lauren Gilmour for the hip-hop video, Dear Human. To Rico, Sean and others Behind the Noise, inspiring young people through music. More recently, to Deborah, Laura, Josh and others in North Lanarkshire, who continue to remind me that true collaboration is possible. From the University, Rosie, Jonathan, Amy and the others who continue to support and inspire me. To On Being and Meditative Story for feeding my soul. To Leah Soweid for reading, referencing, abstracting, encouraging and for going above and beyond. To Nikolina Angelova for thinking and writing with me in the earlier days and for her kindness. To all the communities, all the community members, all of the humans who connected with this research in some way. There are others, so many others, but it's 1:22am GMT on the 16th April 2022, and my Copyedited Manuscript is due, yesterday. Time moves forward, it never moves back. I look outside and, by chance, it's the eve of the Full Moon – a Pink Moon, which I understand to be an illusion. You couldn't make this up.

Time moves back

It's 18:37 BST on the 18th April 2022. I'm sitting in my living room with *Grizzy and the Lemmings* in the background (my three-year-old's current favourite programme described by producer Sean as a modern day *Tom and Jerry* – who's chasing who?). I'm staring at the phone in my hand, shaking, as I try to make sense of the words that are appearing on my small screen. One at a time, one at a time. The internet keeps pushing me news notification after news notification of the same story. It's trying to tell me something. It's *really* trying to tell me something. Review after review after review of a Pulitzer-winning novelist's upcoming book – Jennifer Egan's *The Candy House* – is flooding in, flooding me. I've never heard of her.

Until now.

> **From:** DE ANDRADE Marisa
> **Sent:** 21 April 2022 10:14
> **To:** Jennifer Egan's agents
> **Subject:** my book and Jennifer Egan's The Candy House
>
> Dear Agents,
>
> Reading reviews of Jennifer Egan's *The Candy House* has left me chilled.
>
> In my book, memories are also uploaded and downloaded through an implant and can be seen by others. Memories are similarly owned by a giant corporation that owns all their data and memories and stores them in the Sphere-Blue Drive "to free up headspace for augmented thinking and superior sensing" (or so the marketing slogan says).
>
> One of my characters (a researcher) also keeps wondering how another character (a community member she's researching) can possibly know all of this, and we follow her thoughts through a series of downloaded email and text exchanges and other forms of memory capture devices through DPS (Data Packet Sniffing).
>
> I obviously don't know what other similarities there are between our books as *The Candy House* is only available to the public next week, but it appears we're both writing about collective (un)consciousness, data protection, interconnectedness, and alternative realities. Uncanny.
>
> The key difference is that my book is *not* a work of fiction, but is an academic text. It's narrative *non-fiction* using data from about a decade of my research. It's essentially a methodology book for public health scholars introducing post-qualitative research methods to the discipline with a strong focus on inequalities, and the pathology and medicalisation of mental health.
>
> Routledge commissioned it in 2021 and I submitted my manuscript in January 2022. It's currently in press and will be published in July – Public Health, Humanities and Magical Realism: A Creative-Relational A (routledge.com). The Copyedited Manuscript, which I submitted to my publisher last Saturday, is attached here for your reference. My proofs will arrive any day now.

I felt the need to reach out and let you and Jennifer know. Seeing her thoughts on my computer screen – thoughts so closely aligned with mine – has left me more than a little shaken. Her words also strengthen my academic argument. I'm realising – as I always do when I'm conducting my fieldwork – that we really are a part of something so much bigger than us.

It's 18:37 BST on the 5th May 2022. My publisher's kindly allowed me to add this writing to my Copyedited Manuscript submitted a few weeks ago: "*If you can send me the changes today, I can make them and likely have the proof for your review tomorrow.*"

I think they meant yesterday, I'm hoping we're in different time zones. I need to submit these words as I type them, but what more do I have to say right now?

How do you make sense of two people who've never met – who share cyberspace, a literary device, collective unconscious, humanity – basing their writing on a very similar surreal premise at a parallel time? The Zeitgeist? Coincidence? Human connection? Something else?

I'm now on Chapter 3 of audiobook version of *The Candy House* and I'm in awe of Jennifer's writing. The reviewers are right. It's simply dazzling. Though every so often, I need to pause and process. I can't hear it all at once. It's quite overwhelming. The writing. Particular words, in particular places, particular phrases. It's all so familiar, and I'm not talking plagiarism or copyright or any kind of mind theft other than the kind we share when we pay attention.

I imagine this is what the poet David Whyte means when looking at the hawk, looking back at David, looking back at the hawk, penetrating the essence of humanity. I imagine this is what I was trying to convey somewhere in Chapter 1 of this book.

The "unreal" being inextricably entangled with the "real." Multiple internal realities connecting with an external reality.

This moment, it's happening now, and we've already imagined it and written it.

Figures

Table

1 What's real and unreal in public health?

I saw her for the first time through the windscreen of my terrestrial e-Charge as it cruised towards the infamous Beguile Buildings. As she leaned against a broken bus shelter, her pointy shoulder blades pierced the shattered glass that was more disco ball than protective barrier. She was moving to what appeared to be trance music that only she could hear, her fragile hips occasionally meeting her flicking fingers.

The black skies split open, and her décolletage became a gutter for the downpour. With her eyes closed and a gentle smile dancing on her lips, she warmed me from the inside out. It was two degrees, and she had no coat to speak of except for a flimsy purple scarf draped ceremoniously at her elbows.

I adjusted my coordinates to dodge the pileup of e-Charges that were driving themselves to programmed destinations and slipped into the bus lane. My hazards flashed red as my window rolled down. The street steamed from a week's worth of rain spat from the bellies of dark, pregnant clouds.

She was about a meter in front of me, so I could scan her face for signs of a breakdown. Her edges were surprisingly soft, as if she was dissolving into the grey of the heavens around her. Those black-olive eyes, so alert, attentive, alive.

She looked like Sara. A party girl. Hard to please. Easy on the eye. I found myself drawn to her like a moth to a flame, sensing I was about to get burnt, unable to stop some indescribable force.

I'd arrived in Beguile convinced to find clear confirmation of collective psychosis after analysing The Community's data intensely for seven months. But just seven minutes in, I felt energised. Conflicted. My thinking deconstructed. The story I'd created about this Impoverished Community (dubbed Optimistic Community in policy documents and funding bids)[1] was already being rewritten, my own narrative overwhelmed and revised with it.[2]

I was desperate to speak to her. She must have sensed it. She broke the silence.

"Do you ever see yourself with a bump, swollen and miserable? With a bump, swollen and happy as you rub your unborn child with your nurturing palm?" Her childlike hand circled her concave stomach.

"Pardon?"

"Give it ten years – well, ten years if you believe in time." She looked me straight in the eyes. "A decade, then they'll do away with it."

DOI: 10.4324/9781003196488-1

"Do away with what?"

She was so intense, so assured. Spoke as if delivering a keynote speech, not making chitchat at the bus stop. "Do away with the concept of conception under the Abundant Infertility Act. Gone will be the need to inseminate to safeguard the survival of the human race. Gone will be the need for women to be disadvantaged in the workplace. Gone will be the need for the workplace to be disadvantaged by labour. To be advantaged by the abundance of labour courtesy of procreation by design. The banishing of birth. It'll be hailed as the most progressive policy of its time." Her eyes flickered momentarily at the digital bus schedule as it flashed six minutes to Destination Danda. "You mark my words." She paused as she prophesised.

"Time. Time moves forward. It never moves back. That's [Rule # 1]."[3]

I noticed my fingers pulsing on the dashboard. How could such drivel unnerve me? She was clearly unwell, along with everyone else in The Community – I knew that much from the datasets we'd been analysing. But I hadn't expected this composure. Coherence. Insight[4] even.

"Tell me something: what would you change in your life?" she asked, as if she was the researcher instead of me, her eyes seeing straight into my soul.

***

INTERLUDE – HUMANITIES AND MAGICAL REALISM IN PUBLIC HEALTH

Connecting public health to humanities and magical realism, then claiming that in this unholy alliance lies a "creative and credible" (Daykin et al. 2016)[5] – and necessary – way to research the human experience might, on the surface of it, seem like one universal leap or astral projection too far. At least in this human realm.

About ten years ago, I would've shared your scepticism. Firmly grounded in the principles of public health and receiving funding from organisations that rely on evidence-based science to influence policy and practice, my thinking was straight and narrow.

Then a merger in my academic department got me surrounded by counsellors, psychotherapists, and other applied health social scientists. My horizons widened. I began reading theories on consciousness, the self, psychoanalysis, embodiment, relationality, and affect. Before long, I was trying to make sense of the intersections between anthropology, theology, the philosophy of science, and public health.

My mind exploded.

Most of what I had taught to be true in public health was flipped on its head.

I'd never stopped to consider the nature of reality (ontology) or construction of knowledge (epistemology) in public health. And while power was central to much of my health research, I was studying it in a way that potentially reinforced power *because* I'd never stopped to consider the nature of reality or construction of knowledge.

I sought comfort in the words of the sociologist John Law (Law 2004):[6]

> The powerful (try to) insist that their statements are literal representations of a single reality. "It really is that way", they tell us. "There is no alternative". But those on the receiving end of such homilies learn to read them allegorically. Cynicism, scepticism, the detection of hidden interests, a sense to the ideological, these are the techniques used by subordinates to read through the powerful to the concealed realities that have produced them.

But Law's words equally troubled me. Reviews of his book (now almost two decades old) called *After Method: Mess in Social Science Research* a "controversial," "radical," and "even revolutionary" argument "loved by some but hated by many!" I could hardly imagine public health experts accepting this thesis en masse. Then I remembered that change happens one person at a time. I kept reading and ruminating.

Ironically, it was a physicist, Fritjof Capra, who made me realise that this thesis is not unique to the social – or soft – sciences. The systems theorist connects science, mysticism (or magic), connectivity, and creativity so commonsensically that it surprised me that magical realism wasn't the go-to paradigm for researching the human experience in public health.

Fritjof (Capra and Luisi 2012)[7] tells us,

> "In the human realm, the notion of quality always seems to include references to human experiences, which are subjective aspects. This should not be surprising. Since all qualities arise from processes and patterns of relationships, they will necessarily include subjective elements if these processes and relationships involve human beings. For example, the quality of a human relationship derives largely from subjective mutual experiences."

He goes on to clarify that "to describe and explain the qualities of such subjective experiences within a scientific framework is known as the 'hard problem' of consciousness studies."

In a nutshell, "in the interest of seeking truth," we're trying to understand our reality but keep "getting lost with a slightly dizzy feeling, induced by the arguments going round and round to try and prove what is often posited as the 'common sense' interpretation" (Morgan 2018).[8]

Put simply, our so-called reality is that "the one thing the human mind is incapable of comprehending is itself" (Morgan 2018).[9] Yet we keep going 'round and 'round, trying to prove subjective human experiences in public health through *one* view of reality when "in truth" – is there such a thing? – there are *multiple alternative views of reality.*

So where does this leave us in a discipline committed to evidencing health and well-being at a *population* level? If we're all experiencing different realities at any one time as individuals, how are we supposed to pin down a *collective experience* (is there such a thing?) – and capture it in some way – to come up with policies and practices that will quite literally save lives?

Good questions.

Perhaps the starting point is to "complicate the idea that public health can rely on individual or population level approaches that overlook affective and spatial entanglements" (Barnfield 2016).[10]

Rather than creating a single dominant and coherent narrative, we could start by recording "'accumulations of the moment' . . . in varying quantities and at various times, a combination of 'imagination, humility and courage.'" We could present a few "parallel voices" that simultaneously capture "the excess, loss and chaos" of "ten million stories." Stories that capture the essence of humanity (Speedy 2015).[11]

Flip-flopping back to Law, that messy sociologist working in the discipline of science, technology, and society: "If much of the world is vague, diffuse or unspecific, slippery, emotional, ephemeral, elusive or indistinct, changes like a kaleidoscope, or doesn't really have much of a pattern at all, then where does this leave social science [or public health]? How might we catch some of the realities we are currently missing? Can we know them well? Should we know them?"

More good questions.

I appreciate public health seeks concrete answers, but for now, I invite you to keep reading and to stay open.

I invite you to take solace in "the importance and influence of multiple texts, positions, theories, discourses and actions as sites of affiliation and sharing that unfold across time and into one another like a good conversation" (Holman Jones and Pruyn 2018).[12]

***

"Tell me something: what would you change in your life?" she asked, as if she was the researcher instead of me, her eyes seeing straight into my soul.

I had to answer, that much I was sure of. I looked 'round at the pavements strewn with squashed cans of cider, brown paper bags, cigarette stubs, half-eaten burgers, and energy drinks and thought of my work in public health. The city-view apartment I retired to every night with 500-thread-count, crisp white bedsheets. Something hit the pit of my stomach. Was it fear?

"I would stop gaming the system.[13] Stop being part of the problem." My words appeared to have their own momentum. They welled up, then – without warning, consequence, fact, or my best intention at heart – they released what felt like a violent blow. Without permission, they pulled the trigger on my reality.[14] "What would you change in your life?" I hastened to ask, desperate to cover my vulnerability.

She didn't have think about it. "Nothing. I have everything I need right here, right now. I'm free, connected. So what, some bad stuff's happened to me? So what, I don't know where I'm going next? But here I am, standing in right in front of you, telling you I'm happy, asking you, What are you going to do with your one magical life?"[15]

I believed her. And I didn't know how to answer her. I'd never given purpose that much thought; I was too busy crashing from deadline to deadline. Reports don't write themselves. Funding doesn't just miraculously appear.

In that moment, I wanted to be her. I wanted, so much, to be her. So much to not have a care in the world and to feel. To feel everything as it arrived. To be okay with the not knowing and the arriving and the passing away. To sit with the joys and the sorrows alone and in company and know that no matter where, no matter who, I am never alone. I am always connected by this mysterious empty fullness that this random Community Member embodied as she stood there in the rain with nothing and no one, happy. So, so happy. Deliriously happy.[16]

Then I remembered I was there to fix her. She'd lost her way, lost touch with her reality, and she needed my help.[17]

"What's your name?" I asked gently, as if we were in a therapy room.

"Sara." She smiled mysteriously.

I knew it had to be her.

"Do you want me to show you the way?"

"Excuse me?"

"Do you want me to show you the way to The Futile Forest? You're here to research us, right? I can take you there."

I stared at her, mouth wide open. This human, she knew things. She knew things she couldn't possibly have known. Yes, I was there to research her, to research all of them. But there was no way she could've known that. And we all knew that there wasn't a fake forest or pretend park within miles of this ashtray of a neighbourhood.

"Hop in." My door popped open to the sound of my voice.

Sara slid in beside me, her skeletal frame swallowed by the cushioned bucket seat.

"My e-Charge knows how to get to the Beguile Buildings," I told her as we pulled off into the drizzle. "No need for directions, but I'd like to keep asking you questions, if that's okay . . . ?"

"I'm sure it'll take you there in a straight line as quickly as possible. But why do you want to take the most direct route?" She picked at the chipped blue varnish barely covering her bitten fingernails. "Imagine what you might discover if you take the road less travelled . . ." (Hein 2018)[18]

I thought about the institutional approval I'd just managed to get to come on-site – to enter The Community – after several rounds of ethics applications. Too risky. Too dangerous. Too many unknowns. They're too vulnerable; you're too vulnerable. Not within the remit of the research – there's enough desk-based data to do the analysis; what more do you need to know? Why do you want to see them face-to-face in their own environments?

Did my risk assessment cover having a Community Member in my car? What about my safety? What about hers?

I heard her chuckle. She was looking at me, my face all screwed up, my eyes wide open. I could feel my heart racing as my mind raked through the consequences of my actions.

"Don't panic," she whispered. "This bit isn't real."

"Pardon?"

"You're making this bit up. I'm not actually in the car with you."

"What?"

"Take a left here," she said. The e-Charge carried on in the same direction.

"It only recognises my voice. It won't take instructions from you."

"Tell it to take a left."

"Take a left."

Our perspective had shifted. We were on a bending backstreet heading towards the Beguile Buildings from behind. From above, you'd have seen us meandering through The Wee Chip Bab, Food Bank, Beguile Chemist, Jimmy's Pizza, Pat McTatt Hair, Beguile Park Supermarket, Community Garden, Sheltered Housing, Rest & Recovery Café, and another shop called Munch.

"Another person last month," Sara said, pointing at the high-rises. "We didn't see him very much but noticed when he was gone. Didn't want to carry on anymore, so chose to take life into his own hands and put an end to it." She spoke as if she were reading from the menu of the local takeaway – functional, to the point – but there was a slight quiver in her voice.

"Does that happen often?" I asked gently.

"Suicide?" She gazed at the sky. "More often than you'd think."

She told me how "they" – the people who reported the deaths and tried to make sense of the deaths and tried to fix the people who allegedly didn't have the strength to carry on because they were too unwell – were getting it all wrong.

"Too simple. Too much blame. They just don't get it."

"Don't get what?' I asked, knowing she was trying to tell me I was one of "them."

"The story behind the story. The bigger picture. We get to make choices that work for us."[19]

In the distance, I could see a couple of concrete parking lots with dotted, derelict cars. They weren't on the map I'd been given.

Sara carried on talking, telling me about Lucy, who arrived in The Community from England with her then-boyfriend to make a clean start after a series of abusive relationships down south. "They" had her two children removed from her care. Too unsafe.

This time it would be different, she told herself.

Things were going well. Her new boyfriend found work; they settled into The Community. Then the new boyfriend fell back into using drugs and moved out to protect Lucy. So there she was – alone, isolated – in a new place with no connections, no family nearby, repeating the patterns of her past. Alcohol helped her get up in the morning. Helped her deal with her reality.

"She was close to being another statistic when she found us."

"Found who?" I asked.

"You'll see," Sara smiled. "We're almost there."

"Almost where?"

"You'll see. It's out of this world."

The way Sara was bigging this up, I half-expected a Jumanji-style forest emerging from the slabs just a few hundred meters in front of my eyes.

"And then there's Mary, who was born in Beguile but spent most of her childhood moving from one place to another with her mum and sister, running away from her violent dad. She liked school and left to study at college, but her close relative got sick, really sick, and didn't make it. This hit Mary hard. So, so hard. She dropped out. One night she met a guy, and it was love at first sight. He was everything she'd never had. They moved in together quickly – like matching eternity bracelets quickly – within months of meeting. He was the one. Sure, he drank a lot and took quite a bit of drugs, but she stayed strong and didn't get pulled into his addictions. Until the battering began . . . stop here . . ."

"Here?" We'd driven through the first of the two car parks and were about 400 meters from a fire escape route that everyone knew didn't stand a chance of saving lives in these tower blocks if someone left their fry-up on for too long. Something to do with cladding. Defective materials.

"Follow me." I watched Sara as she swaggered to what looked like a lift camouflaged in concrete. I was shaking, I realised, as I looked up at wispy white clouds crossing over one another in an endless blue sky. The storm had passed.

I'd read her case notes so knew everything about Sara. More than that, we'd completed our analysis, so I knew everything about everyone like her in The Community. I knew what was wrong with them. They'd all had a "mental health issue." All had taken part in a Clinical Trial. They'd all, at some point, been on antidepressants or another type of medication, but their circumstances and health outcomes remain unchanged. They all continued to be individually and collectively morose and overindulging in what we, the Public Health Experts, call Health-Damaging Behaviours – smoking, drinking, eating junk food, and so on.

Everything we'd tried hadn't worked.[20] The Community was deemed to be a Public Health Disaster. We, the Public Health Experts, had been brought in to conduct the Straightforward Inane Lucid Liability (SILLY) Clinical Trial from our offices and labs – all virtually conducted from the comfort of homes since The Final Lockdown – armed with a rigorous research design with all the hallmarks of a proper, credible, scientific study.

We quickly discovered members in The Community had all gone mad. Some of them were claiming a pine marten[21] (a sort of weasel – I didn't know what this was either) was making them feel well. Others were seeking comfort and health in poetry.

We contemplated bringing a team of psychiatric nurses into The Community to assess for collective psychosis, especially when we encountered two members in The Community conducting their own study (they were not even researchers!) with the silliest of research questions: Is a poem or a pine marten better for your mental health?

It was all unprecedented. I felt compelled to do something. To know for myself. What I was doing – stepping into The Community with actual human contact – was arguably madder than their communal madness. But I couldn't stop myself.

As I found myself following Sara, doing what I'd been told, I wondered why it was I who was quivering. Why wasn't she the embodiment of the destructive force detailed in our findings? Why wasn't she confused? Jittery? Vulnerable?

Why was I the bag of nerves? As if she'd taken a pair of pinking shears to the very tips of my nerve endings and tickled them with jagged, zigzagged teeth sharp enough to cut right through me?[22]

We stepped into the clandestine elevator. Took it to the 212th floor of a building shaped like a ginormous, bulbous pear. As we ascended, Sara resumed her story.

"So for years, Mary stayed with him and tried to stay out of drinks and drugs and all the things that shaped her boyfriend's life. Easier said than done. Oh, did I mention she fell pregnant fourteen weeks after meeting him, which made getting away from him almost impossible? You couldn't make this up. Eventually, the drug beatings got so bad that the police got involved. The violence got worse, and he was sentenced for stabbing someone who owed him money. It was all pretty grim. By this point she had a one-year-old."

Sara took a breath as we passed floor 100. Something unsettling was coming. I could feel it.

"While he was in jail, Mary somehow got caught up in carrying on his business of selling drugs. She needed the cash to keep her baby alive. Then, slowly, she started taking drugs herself. Just a little at the start, but soon she was on a slippery slope. One day, she went to her doctor for help. They asked her all sorts of questions, sent her to an addiction service, did psychiatric assessments – that confirmed she wasn't mad – but they said if she didn't get her act together quickly, her child would get taken out of her care."

I started feeling nauseous. This story. This never-ending elevator ride. These four solid walls that were fast becoming a cell. We were only at 161. She carried on.

"She was scared to death, doing everything she could to sort her life out, but by this point she'd been spat out of the services because there really wasn't anything wrong with her. Before long, she was addicted to crack and heroin, and there was no way she was going back for help. All she remembered them saying was her child was going to get taken away from her, so she sat in silence, trying to sort her own stuff out, trying to take care of herself and her toddler between the highs and lows.

"After her boyfriend was released from jail, he seriously hurt Mary again – this time to her back – and the police were called. Because he was tagged, she was taken away from the crime scene. Luckily, her kid was at a friend's house. Then things went from bad to worse. Legal highs became her drug of choice. She started getting bouts of paranoia and proper aggression. She got violent."

Was this ever going to end? I felt dizzy, as if I was having an out-of-body experience. 200.

"Eventually, Mary ran away to stay with someone in her family. They're helping look after her kid. An agency helped her get supported accommodation, but her ex-boyfriend still found her and started harassing her. Now *he* was threatening to take her kid away from her. She moved to another place in recovery, started feeling a better about her future. She wants to support women who've gone through some of what she had gone through. She knows she has to stick to the recovery programme, and she knows what she needs to study to work with people in The Community."[23]

Ping. 212. Stale air gushed in. I'd never been so pleased by pollution. Perspective is everything.

I looked down at the bulging base of a building that had tapered at the top to reveal a stalk, a farther structure almost imperceptible to the naked eye from below. Sara swiped a card, and the stem slid open to expose a second lift door.

"Come on, we're almost there." I shuffled in. There was no going back now.

Up, up, up we went to the very tip of the stalk.

"Mary feels very safe here – and in her temporary accommodation – but she knows it's only for now. She wants her own place, but there are no rentals in her budget. She wants to get out into The Community and get stuck into groups and do things that'll make her feel alive again – as if she's not alone – but there's no chance. She's scared for her safety. Now she's been offered a tenancy in another part of the UK, so she's heading off soon. New place, new people, new beginning . . . again. Always change, never safe in one place. She has no choice, really. She's really happy about it, mind you. She's tough. Hopeful. She's been through so much."

Ping.

"Are you ready for this?" she smiled warmly. The doors parted, and the sun poured in.

I rubbed my eyes, convinced they were playing tricks on me. This couldn't be real.

"Welcome to The Futile Forest."[24]

***

INTERLUDE – FINDINGS, FACTS, FABRICATIONS, AND SOUL FOOD

You're at a crossroads now, reader, much like the anonymous researcher in this *writing*.

So you're – we're – at a crossroads now, reader.

Do you believe what you're seeing in front of you even though, like the anonymous researcher, you're convinced your eyes are playing tricks on you and, you believe, The Futile Forest couldn't possibly be real?

Or do you – we – believe Sara and accept her reality for what she says it truly is?

Your dilemma is even more complex than mine as, I suspect, your decision-making will be influenced by an awareness that I'm drawing on the (speculative) humanities rather than the (factual) empirical approaches of the natural sciences.

Also, if you research or work in public health (and there's a strong chance you do as you're the target audience of this book), then chances are you're probably struggling to take much of this seriously anyway. We don't tend to mix the joys of reading or writing creative prose or poetry with the business of reading or writing proper, rigorous, academic, scientific publications (Law 2004).

As Victoria Foster (Foster 2016)[25] muses in her book *Collaborative Arts-based Research for Social Justice*, "arts-based methods have ineffable, 'magical' qualities," so how do we know "the extent to which 'truths' can be communicated through this [sort of] razzle dazzle . . . ?"

After all, "ascribing meaning to others' experiences often requires a cautious touch so as not to lose the 'magic' that the artistic work produces and so as not to privilege the researchers' (already privileged) position. Both the artistic work and the accompanying explanations produced through arts-based inquiry need to promote conversation that enables us to 'see more deeply'" (Foster 2016).[26]

More deeply into what? I find myself wondering.

The first word that comes to mind is the *soul*.

I remember reading about Charlotte Salomon's work "as an example of how art can plumb the depths of the personal soul while inciting others to creative action" (McNiff 2008).[27]

Art, quite literally, saved her life:

> *Charlotte Salomon was twenty-three years old in 1940 when she made a painting of her face – a nameless, stateless, Jewish face. At the time, she was living as a refugee from Nazism in Villefranche on the French Riviera, and she had just made a startling discovery: that eight members of her family, one by one, over the years, had committed suicide. With this traumatic revelation in mind, she arrived at what she called "The question: whether to take her own life or to undertake something eccentric and mad." Something "eccentric and mad" turned out to be an artwork in over seven hundred scenes, painted during one year (1941–1942), enriched by dialogues, soliloquies, and musical references, arranged into acts and scenes, and titled "Life? Or Theater? An Operetta." This massive artwork recounted the story of her Berlin Jewish family from World War I up to the day in 1941 when she decided to paint her life rather than to take it, then sat down by the Mediterranean "and saw deep into the heart of humankind."*[28]

So poignant. To paint your life rather than to take it. To sit surrounded by war and pain and trauma and to take it in. Fully. Then to transform that war and pain and trauma into an imaginative manifestation of what you're feeling on the inside, to reflect what is happening on the outside. Or to take what is happening on the outside in so that you can feel it on the inside.

Inside, outside. Internal reality, external reality.

It's all connected.

Charlotte connected with what Capra would call "the breath of life" or "spirit," "a way of being that flows from a profound experience of reality, which is known as 'mystical', 'religious' or 'spiritual' experience" (Capra and Luisi 2012).[29]

Now let's just pause for a moment and acknowledge that spirituality[30] isn't something that Western public health practitioners and scholars tend to feel particularly comfortable with as a collective – unless we're trying to measure it on a scale in relation to health outcomes.

Speaking about the "soul" in health policy appears to "raise some eyebrows or cause you to shift a bit in your seat" (Hustedde 1998).[31] Some public health researchers – and I include my earlier self in this cohort – shy away from the term *spirituality* as they do not view it as legitimate. Others interpret it as a means to conceal more significant issues (Driver 2010).

Through a critical lens, it's perceived by some as exploitative and used by organisations for instrumental gain (Cook 2004). Alternatively, it's framed as "psychological coercion."[32] A distraction from the structural origins of health inequalities (Smith and Schrecker 2015) and efforts to address the health impact of corporate power (Friedli 2013).

Yes, speaking about spirituality appears to be deeply discomforting in health policy circles in the West, particularly the UK, even though the principles of asset-based working, person-centred care, compassion, and empathy are explicit in health and social care discourses, policies, and practices. In Scotland, where health is improving less rapidly than in any other country in Europe, efforts are focused on reducing a persistent health inequalities gap. Health practitioners are obliged – by laws, such as the Community Empowerment Act – to engage and "empower" the most disadvantaged in our society by mobilising their skills and knowledge and making them less reliant on public services (Sigerson and Gruer 2011).

Some scholars insist there is no evidence that these "soft" approaches can explain and tackle health inequalities, a key reason for promoting them in the first place. Others go one step further, asserting that their implementation in deprived communities contributes to social abjection by stigmatising the poor (Tyler 2013). This, according to some, is propagated through "a common evangelical language" (Stearn and Friedli 2013) speaking to "something within the spirit of individuals living within deprived communities that needs healed" (Scottish Community Development Centre 2011).[33]

Then there are reflections on what they perceive to be a paradox of epidemiology: "As material inequalities grow, so the pursuit of non-material explanations* for health outcomes proliferates" (Friedli 2013).[34]

* Such touchy-feely enlightenments include "the familiar roll-call of self-esteem, aspiration, confidence, optimism, sense of coherence, meaning and purpose, the so-called intangible assets such as knowledge, skills, wisdom and culture, and key features of social capital: social networks, reciprocity, mutual aid and collective efficacy" (Friedli 2013).[35]

---

* I'd call this a story, but then, maybe, you'd think it was all made-up. Not true. I'd call this my research findings, but then, maybe, you'd think I was reporting facts from my fieldwork. True, to some extent, but I couldn't begin to convey with words what actually happened in the field that day in a way that would do justice to what actually happened in the field on that day. You would've had to have been there with me in that moment. Sensed what I was sensing in that moment. The best I can do is try to recreate that moment in some way with the rather-limited medium of the written word. This is a book, after all, and for me to be taken seriously as a scholar, I need to publish.

Adding spirituality to this list will not make some public health experts happy, and their arguments need to be taken seriously, given insurmountable global inequalities. Though my fieldwork sparked the idea that spirituality is embedded in popular, contemporary health policies advocating the use of bottom-up, community-led, asset-based approaches (de Andrade and Angelova 2017).[36] Some unworldly, transcendent essence was always there when I engaged with community members and health workers, hidden behind more palatable expressions such as positive psychology and salutogenesis, sometimes dressed up in more savoury terms, such as *sense of coherence* and *resilience*.

As I read critiques of the "evangelical zeal" of asset-based approaches in health policy discourses and understood more about why they are denounced by some as "a significant a feature of conditionality in the lives of those who are poor as going to church once was" (Friedli and Stearn 2015), my mind drifted to the origins of the approach.

The story of spirituality in public health arguably began in the concentration camps during the Second World War, when Viktor Frankl – psychiatrist, neurologist, and prisoner – reflected on "the last of human freedoms." By doing this, he claimed to discover meaning in life. The school of logotherapy he founded, which aimed to carry out an existential analysis of a person, was grounded in hope. A belief that we can finding meaning in life and in our suffering regardless of our circumstances in three different ways: By creating something or doing something for someone. By experiencing something or meeting someone who affects you. And by the way we think about and work with life's inevitable suffering (Frankl 1984).

Extensive research claims to have validated Frankl's theories on the spiritual elements of humanity using quantitative measures to capture personal meaning (for example through the Personal Meaning Profile and Life Regard Index) and qualitative measures (through personal narratives) (Wong and Fry 1998).

But is it possible to "validate the feels"? I wonder (de Andrade 2017).[37]

Man's Search for Meaning, written by the holocaust survivor, inspired Anton Antonovsky's work on salutogenesis focusing on the determinants of health rather than the determinants of illness (Antonovsky 1996). Asset-based approaches drew on this model to highlight the importance of working with the capacities and resources that people already have when developing services and interventions to improve community health and well-being (Rippon and Hopkins 2015; Foot 2012).

Asset-based approaches. That's how I stumbled into another story that's being told here, while walking the streets of "disadvantaged" communities, speaking to so-called hard-to-reach communities applying asset-based approaches in an alarmingly reductionist way.

I went in to The Community thinking I could measure humanistic aspects related to their health and well-being through a formulaic framework. I came out compelled to accept and embrace "direct, non-intellectual experience[s] of reality in moments of heightened aliveness" – "mystical experience[s]" with "a profound sense of connectedness, of belonging to the cosmos as a whole." I came out "incapable" of "adequately" expressing these moments "in words or concepts." I came out "with a deep sense of awe and wonder together with a feeling of great humility" (Capra and Luisi 2012).[38]

I could no longer *do* public health research the way I was taught, the way I used to see it, the way I used to interpret it. I sensed a bold, reflexive shift towards a critical view of "self" and "other," an uncovering and retelling of our stories within the academy and beyond, which felt like a tentative first step in attending to systemic issues in a different way.

The experience rendered me vulnerable, but also connected to myself, "others," and the world at large. Some words etched on the pavement of a walk along the John Muir Way told me I was on a meaningful track: "When we try to pick out anything by itself, we find it hitched to everything else in the universe (Muir 1911)."[39]

***

"Welcome to The Futile Forest."

She stepped into some sort of make-believe sanctuary. It had to be a mock-up – flora and fauna were things of the past – but I'd never seen a replica parkland or fake spot of nature of this kind in This World.

Hovering in the clouds, perched near the stars. A circular green space of epic proportions exposed to the elements.

"If you were in a helicopter, you'd make out its perfect symmetry from above," Sara said matter-of-factly. "Twelve spokes on a wheel, each segment a perfect slice of nature. In the middle, a big Bodhi tree[40] that sheds leaves like a snake sheds skins but never dies. Just constant renewal, as long as there's enough water in its roots."

I closed my eyes, breathed in the crisp sunset. The air had the smell of starting over. And wet wild mushrooms. I spotted one looking like a little palm tree with a sombrero instead of leaves. Another was shaped like an oversized golf tee, I noticed as we walked slowly. Almost meditatively.

"Take your time," she advised. "There's a lot to take in."

I opened my mouth to say something, anything, but there were no words. I couldn't get my thoughts and memories in order. They were uncharacteristically scattered. Ping-ponging between flashbacks so real and intense the one second, so illusionary and fleeting the next, reality suspended somewhere in the middle.

What was real and what wasn't real about meeting Sara? I mentally murmured to a great oak still soaking up the afternoon's downpour. A single swallow created a fine shower as it flew from branch to twig then took off like a shuttlecock to join a second swallow in the sky. Together, two swallows turned to salmon swimming upstream in unison.

I blinked several times to bring my eyes back to the reality of that present moment. *Those are birds. Birds. Not fish. Birds, not fish.* More mind ramblings.

Don't get too close to participants—that was one of the rules. Just get close enough to get them to open up to you, closer still to extract data. And eject. Get away from the person. Get away from The Community.

And here I was, up close and personal, feeling connected. Creative. Relational.

I stepped on to damp blades that, for a moment, turned to razors under my feet, and focused my attention on a path a woodchuck had carved, kicking small bits of timber. Sara strolled beside me. I was too scared to look at her again, but I did and was blinded by a light so fierce and intense that for a moment I became the sunset.

Then the darkness returned.

She shook me to my core. I knew there was no going back. I felt connected to her on some inexplicable level that maybe I'd spend the rest of my days trying to explain to myself.

There's no way I can explain it to others, I thought. I'm not even going to try.

Sara stopped to watch a spider doing bondage with a fly in the silkiest of ropes, right beside a bush of purple pincushions scratching the belly of a bee. She smiled as if thistles were her favourite. As if she loved how their lavender shade made them appear to be gentle even though they were spiky by nature.

Then she delicately picked burnt-orange and white petals from a flower with a mane, its lion face a pursed green tomato.

I thought about how effortless she was with her nonsense utterings. Spouting prophesies so matter-of-factly, clearly believing in the madness that poured from her mouth. Or maybe she'd mastered the art of lying to the extent that she could trick her own mind into believing she was telling the truth. I wasn't sure yet.

A butterfly landed on the grass. Its furry, velvet royal blue eyes stared me out. I felt as if The Futile Forest was watching me. The insects. Were there CCTV cameras hidden in trees, their wooden eyeballs carved into trunks?

I suddenly felt paranoid.

The ones on the two rows of eight symmetrically aligned Cigarette Trees looked particularly demonic. Red rings 'round black pupils etched into thin white bark covered in layers of wood-chipped wallpaper. I imagined you could peel off layer upon layer, the one underneath becoming yellower. More nicotine-stained. Little roll-ups fell to the earth.

I felt like I was getting closer to something. My mind was no clearer, but I felt alive. Confused, but alive. Sleepwalking through life, jumping from theory to thesis. All this no longer seemed possible.

A bumble bee buzzed past my ear and settled in a flower masquerading as a gramophone.

We turned right into the thick of the forest leading to a Bodhi tree where Sara spread herself across the bench beneath it, stomach to the heavens. The sun squinted through leaves like a kaleidoscope. A single white feather floated towards her face as the winds spoke over one another.

Yes, I thought as my phone started ringing, *I've taken my first step on this path, and there is no going back.*

My phone rang out. Seconds later, it rang again. And again. I was annoyed at myself for not turning it on silent. This was not a time for disruptions from the real world.

I reached to turn it off, then saw the name flashing on my screen.

My hands trembled. Professor Ebba from the Upper Echelons of The Institution (Jackson and Mazzei 2012).[41] I would never get a call from her unless . . . unless . . .

This had to be serious.

Sara caught the feather between her left thumb and forefinger and gently blew it away as I cleared my throat.

"Hello, Professor Ebba," I said with a wavering voice.

***

INTERLUDE – CRITICAL REALISM MEETS MAGICAL REALISM

It's 3:00 a.m., and I can't sleep. Something is stirring inside me as I write this truthful tale of magical realism. Something is bothering me.

I can't deny that as I'm writing this, I'm critical. Critical of what I'm writing. Critical of the external environment and all its inequities.

I can't deny that critical realism[42] has comforted me in some way. Knowing that there is an objective reality out there (for example, social, commercial, and political determinants of health) to contextualise the pain and trauma that comes with disparities in our existence as humans on this planet, at this time.

So why am I messing about with the literary genre of magical realism in the discipline of public health – a style of writing with a name that suggests fiction, fantasy, and falsehood?

Well, for starters, the name is deceptive as "the magic in magic realism has deep roots in the real."[43] The characters (community members, researcher[s], academics, funder[s]) are ordinary people doing ordinary things (eating, drinking, hanging out, working, or trying to survive) in familiar places (bus stops, vehicles, high-rise buildings, gardens). They exist in real-world surroundings.

But something doesn't quite make sense. Certain circumstances or incidents are a bit odd. Irrational even. You'd think the narrator would point out the obvious and say, "Hey, guys, you know that isn't logical? You know you can't turn the rooftop of a high-rise building in a disadvantaged neighbourhood into some sort of wannabe garden of Eden?"

But no. The narrator is totally on board with it all. Speaks very matter-of-factly. Accepts reality for what it truly appears to be. There's no questioning of the surreal. Only acceptance.

Magical realism also swirls about in the boundless coil of a time warp. There's no linearity. The narrative shifts rapidly without any warning. The reader is whisked into supernatural states of being, and signs from the universe and super-powers, such as mind reading and fortune-telling, prevail. It isn't uncommon for fables and ritualistic entities, such as forest guardians and spiritual ancestors, to materialise.

All these literary devices are intentionally grounded in real-world, historical, and social contexts.[44] The magical in the made-up world bumps up against what I consider to be ontological certainties in the world we live in to allow for a deep dive into structural issues and human traits such as poverty, inequalities, racism, abuse, prejudice, condemnation, oppression, and superiority.

This could be conceptualised as the "unreal" being inextricably entangled with the "real." Multiple internal realities connecting with an external reality.

But how to bring all these worlds and realities together?

I sense there's an answer out there – or in here – but right now, I can't figure out what it is or where it is. Instead, I start listening to a podcast, *Meditative Story*. I've become very fond of it; it is beautiful, combining "human stories with meditation prompts embedded into the storylines – all surrounded by breath-taking music."[45]

I get instantly drawn into a captivating episode narrated by the Welsh poet David Whyte. I'd never heard of him before but know now he's written ten volumes of poetry and four of prose, including the bestselling *The Heart Aroused: Poetry and the Preservation of the Soul in Corporate America.*[46]

"I'm 'quietly unravelling,'" he says barely louder than a whisper. He speaks of being "traumatised by beauty," "barely holding on to the fixed sanity" he's brought with him, "insulated aloneness."

His words pique me.

The hours pass. I toss and I turn. I can't shake the image of a beautiful trauma. What does he mean by this curious oxymoron?

What happens when he meets that "unblinking, unmoving guardian to the secret of [his] future life"?

Now I'm wide awake, transcribing the podcast verbatim.[47] Intrigued. It's day-break, and I'm waiting for my toddler to wake me. Life feels still. Brimming. Full of possibilities.

For a moment, I believe this poet I've never heard of is talking to me, me and only me, as he vividly recalls a life-changing magical encounter with a majestic Galapagos hawk staring him square in the eyes:

> *I stop and I stare back. I am looking into the essence of hawkness in the world. I am looking straight into the well and the depth of its eyes. I am looking at that corner of creation which laughs at any manufactured name we have given it. It is hawkness itself. Time stops its linear procession and begins to radiate from where I stand. I feel simultaneously a physical body unravelling in the sense of revelation all at the same time.*

And then his realisation, which I realise captures the essence of what I'm saying in Measuring Humanity,[48] and my realisation that he is speaking to us all:

> *The surprise in the revelation is that I have the experience of the hawk looking just as deeply into that corner of creation that I occupy in my humanity. But it is looking*

straight beneath any surface personality. Any David Whyte-ness and straight to another, unnameable foundation that I am just beginning to understand.

Later in the episode, he wonders whether the famous artist William Blake – "a poet and engraver originally considered insane and cast aside by his peers but now recognized as one of the greatest contributors to English language and art"[49] – actually spoke with the angels or whether it was a "metaphor that he stood in conversation with worlds beyond our own." Are there "invisible worlds larger than our own"? Is there "another source of help larger than us in the world"?[50]

I find myself having an internal debate about whether this is too far-fetched. Too woo-woo.

Insane is such a charged word. Mad ones with their cryptic communication, abstract art, and moments of connection in nature with spirit animals and spiritual guides.

No wonder science is separated from the arts and humanities. Being human is separated from evidence-based science.

A thesis is solidifying and then shape-shifting. To deepen my inquiry, I do some fire walking, meditation, yoga, and healing dance practices like the ones some Community Members have told me about. I attend a shamanic drumming circle.

Swirl and swirl together, our fingers weaved together. Breathing our being in a sphere of love. Our connection is deep, and the swirl continues.[51]

It's a week later now, a full moon in Aquarius. A blue moon – as in once in a blue moon – and again I'm moved by the tides and drawn to my laptop in the middle of the night.

As I stare at this stunning cosmological specimen, I realise that I've been here before. This moment, I've already written it. I've already submitted it to my publisher, Routledge, in November 2020. It's been accepted for publication, and my manuscript is due in six months.

This moment, it's happening now, and I've already imagined it and written it, in the form of a book proposal, nine months ago:

1.1 Statement of aims

1.1.1 What is my book about?

Imagine public health is on the cusp of a paradigm shift and about to take the words of Pablo Picasso quite literally: "*Everything you can imagine is real.*"[52] Imagine it is your task to sift through and make sense of what public health research, policy, and practice says is real (evidence, objectivity, validity, truth) and unreal (opinion, subjectivity, weakness, falsehood) in this contradictory, liminal space of science and fiction.

This is what happens to the author of this book one sleepless night on the eve of the Flower Supermoon one day in May in The Future. She becomes transparent. A fluid being lodged between two epistemic bubbles, stuck between a pair of conflicting paradigms.

On one side stands the heavyweight – public health – supported by evidence-based "certainties" and a multitude of indicators that cover "*the full spectrum of what we understand public health to be, and what we can realistically measure at the moment*" (Office for Health Improvement and Disparities 2013).

On the other, a meagre imposter – humanities and arts – trying to capture the intangible aspects of the human experience and make them more meaningful rather than measurable. Trying to embrace all the uncertainties and complexity of being human to arrive at the answer(s) that public health seeks.

A phantom figure, she steps into the abyss and tries to bridge this gap, toing and froing, trying to make sense of reality (well aware that she isn't real herself), seeking to *Measure Humanity* through the mechanism of magical realism.

She convinces herself it's going well, and even manages to hoodwink leading medical and public health editors and journals. But something doesn't quite feel right.

In her quest to (simply) measure (complex) person-centred and community- or asset-based health care in a meaningful way, she realises she's become less human. Her efforts to objectify the subjective – to capture and categorise what could be defined as comparable moments of heartfelt emotion for measurement purposes – have become similarly reductionist and simplistic.

She realises she's tried to shoehorn similar lived experiences into the same (box) to appease the academy, funders, health bodies, and policymakers.

Meanwhile, the humans she's engaged with on the margins through humanities and arts-informed methods – ethnic minorities, the Deaf community, "those struggling with mental health" (aren't we all?) or living in disadvantaged communities – have somehow been muted. On the surface of it, their voices appear to be heard and represented in health research, policy, and practice. In "reality," their lives remain unaffected and impoverished.

She embarks on a creative mission to untangle and demystify what happens when individual lived, embodied, and even unsubconscious experiences of inequality collide with the system.

She listens to personal stories from "vulnerable" populations (even though the word *vulnerable* makes her shudder), who are suffering most from isolation, poverty, and poor health outcomes compounded by socio-economic threats (Macintyre et al. 2018; Collins 2016).

She sees how their life circumstances are multifaceted and affected by power, context, and relationships (Patel et al. 2018; Katz et al. 2019; Tough, Siegrist, and Fekete 2017).

Floating between science and "fiction," flip-flopping between traditional and alternative post-qualitative, arts-informed methodologies as she critically analyses her datasets, she reflects on her own values and emotions as an "objective" researcher in public health.

This book is drawn from about ten years of researching tobacco control, inequalities, and the system from the top down (think power, regulation and oppression) and studying the well-being of marginalised communities from the bottom up (think creativity, social movements, and freedom).

Is it possible and ethical to be unaffected by and distant from public health data and research "participants"? What is the role researchers play in maintaining or even exacerbating inequalities? How can creative and individualistic approaches challenge structural causes of inequality and public health elitism?

How can we make the system – and public health – more human?

Notes

1 This story is imaginatively informed by an Aspiring Communities project funded by the European Social Fund through the Scottish government in partnership with the charity Bethany Christian Trust.

2 My writing here is influenced by Daniel White's reflection on affect's "methodological challenges and its ontological spirit." In particular, I'm lured by this description: "Even so, the question of affect's role as an intensity that variously energizes, contradicts, deconstructs, and overwhelms the narratives through which we live nonetheless serves as a driving force in much of their work" (White 2017) (page 178).

3 I'm pulled towards the idea of this story floating in a liminal space. From the Latin *limens*, meaning threshold, a state of being that is "neither one thing nor another; or maybe both; or neither here nor there; or maybe nowhere . . . 'betwixt and between' recognized fixed points in the space-time of structural classification" (Turner 1967) (page 96).

4 In mental health, *insight* is a clinical term used to describe "a correct attitude to a morbid change in oneself . . . the realisation that the illness is mental . . . to see ourselves as others see us" (Lewis 1934). For example, the insight to know that one is being psychotic. Neil Allen (Allen 2009) notes, "Not only does insight have different meanings; there are also different tests for measuring it. There is the Insight and Treatment Attitude Questionnaire; the Scale to Assess Unawareness of Mental Disorder; the Insight Scale; Beck's Cognitive Insight Scale; and Birchwood's Insight Scale. Not to mention David's Schedule for the Assessment of Insight. Høyer goes so far as to argue that the content of these tests is virtually meaningless: '[T]hose agreeing with their treating psychiatrist have insight, those who disagree have not'" (page 165).

5 Page 123.

6 Page 89.

7 Page 369.

8 Page 1.

9 Ibid.

10 Ibid.

11 Page 32.

12 Page 11.

13 I'm inspired by Toby Lowe's critical thinking on "target based performance management" that creates perfect conditions for gaming (Lowe and Wilson 2017).

14 Daniel White's words on affect once again spring to mind (White 2017).

15 Channelling Mary Oliver's poem "The Summer Day," originally published in 1992.

16 I'm beginning to reflect on community members with (mental) health issues or so-called problems as "embodied emotion work." What does it feel like to be well or unwell? How are expressions of being (un)well manifested in the body as feelings or emotions, alongside corporeal practices linked to promoting or reducing well-being? Amy Chandler's work on embodiment and self-injury (Chandler 2012) is with me.

17 I'm also thinking about the power and pathology inherent in (mental) (ill) health. Who decides if someone is well or unwell? Who decides what is "true" and "fixable" for them?

18 Page 6. I'm reflecting on the nonlinearity of my research journey and how this jars with "mainstream qualitative research [that] tacitly assumes that researchers strive to create clear, linear, internally coherent, and meaningful texts that adhere to a basic structure. It also assumes that researchers are subjects, stable narrators, who can articulate phenomena unambiguously and that the participants who are described display a similar level of fixity and are organized according to a structure."

19 Sara's reflections of suicide in the community align with Amy Chandler's work in critical suicide studies, which seeks "to counter the limitations of dominant quantitative, positivist, and pathologising approaches" and "develop alternative readings of suicide through rigorous research that draws on the humanities and social sciences." Through this lens, suicide is a "voluntary rather than pathological act" and "a product of cultural forces situated outside the individual" (Chandler, Cover, and Fitzpatrick 2022) (page 2).

20 This is informed by Lynne Friedli's critique of asset-based community development approaches being ineffective and reinforcing structural issues and propping up the institutions that perpetuate inequalities (Friedli 2013).

21 A community worker in one of my studies once told me that seeing pine martens in nature and being immersed in green spaces made them feel alive. Healthier. More connected to life. They said this was the best antidepressant for them. It's a powerful image that's stayed with me ever since.

22 The image of emotional projection comes to mind. Quoting Sarah Ahmed and Ruth Behar, Victoria Foster notes, '"Emotion has been projected into the bodies of others', who are then pathologised as a result (Ahmed 2004; Foster 2016) (page 170), [and] such a projection also 'works to conceal the emotional wrenching ways in which we attain knowledge of others and ourselves'" (Ruth 2008; Foster 2016) (page 63).

23 Sara's, Lucy's, Mary's, and the other life stories integrated into this narrative are informed by the lived experiences encountered and retold to me by community workers in the field. These are not fabrications of reality. Names and all identifying information have been anonymised and adapted for confidentiality.

24 The conceptualisation of The Futile Forest came from an evaluation of the Wild Ways Well approach funded by The Conservation Volunteers (TCV). It sought to explore the use of the outdoor environment and connection with nature to improve health and well-being and to support and enhance individual and community assets. Early evaluations attempted to use traditional quantitative and qualitative approaches to objectively measure attributes such as social trust in green spaces, but soon community evaluators realised the limitations of these approaches. When interviewed, they stressed their need "to work on the existing evidence" showing the impact of nature "to move mental health issues" but wondered how you "prove" this. How do you build the evidence base in this way? What does evidence mean in this situation? And how do you prove that your journey through improved mental health was linked to being outdoors?

25 Page 74.

26 Page 72, quoting (Cahnmann-Taylor and Siegesmund 2008).

27 Page 38.

28 Charlotte Salomon, Jewish Women's Archive: https://jwa.org/encyclopedia/article/salomon-charlotte (Felstiner Lowenthal 1999).

29 Page 277.

30 Christopher Cook (Cook 2004), having reviewed a number of ways of defining *spirituality*, has drawn up the following definition to express its essence: "Spirituality is a distinctive, potentially creative and universal dimension of human experience arising both within the inner subjective awareness of individuals and within communities, social groups and traditions. It may be experienced as relationship with that which is intimately 'inner', immanent and personal, within the self and others, and/or as relationship with that which is wholly 'other', transcendent and beyond the self. It

is experienced as being of fundamental or ultimate importance and is thus concerned with matters of meaning and purpose in life, truth and values" (page 8).

31 Page 153.
32 From the Centre for Medical Humanities blog (Stearn and Friedli 2013).
33 Page 3.
34 Page 131.
35 Page 132.
36 Asset-based approaches value the assets, capacities, and resources that people already have. In contrast to deficit models which explore the *needs* of community, asset-based approaches create conditions for health by strengthening the *assets* of individuals and communities, with *assets* defined as any factors or resources which have an impact on maintaining and sustaining health and well-being on individual, community, and structural levels (see paper for extensive definitions and citations).
37 "Validating the Feels" (https://measuringhumanity.org/validating-the-feels) is a concept that emerged during my Measuring Humanity research process (more on this soon) and was promoted by Audit Scotland – the country's public service watchdog responsible for checking public money is spent efficiently and effectively across 227 public bodies, including central government, councils, NHS bodies, joint integration boards, and further education colleges. They drew inspiration from Measuring Humanity to help them understand and develop ways of assessing where community engagement was working well so it could be audited. The project raised tough questions for the auditor about how we "measure humanity" and cocreate value in public services by accounting for community members' lived experiences. Audit Scotland concluded, "Quantitative data will not give sufficient understanding of the quality of community engagement. A narrative behind each Participation Request via the Community Empowerment is now required to appreciate how community engagement is approached by an organisation."
38 Page 278.
39 These are the words of John Muir, the founder of modern conservation (Muir 1911).
40 The tree of awakening in Buddhism. Buddha is believed to have spent an entire week in front of it, attaining enlightenment.
41 Page 8. Here I'm drawing inspiration from Spivak when thinking about marginality and how power and knowledge are constructed in the academy. According to Alecia Jackson and Lisa Mazzei, "Spivak relies on Foucault's concept of power/knowledge to position the teaching machine (the university) as a vehicle of power/knowledge that seeks to locate and define what counts as authentic inhabitants of the margin. Thus we learn from both Foucault and Spivak how the center (the academy) positions and defines marginality through its constitution of the subject."
42 Philosophical thinking that differentiates between the "real" world (which can't be observed, as it exists autonomously from human perceptions and theories) and the "observable" world (constructed through our perspectives and experiences). This is a bit of a halfway house between positivism and interpretivism. The thinking calls for the separation of reality (ontology) and epistemology (knowledge) (Archer et al. 1998).
43 This is a quote from renowned magical realist author Salmon Rushdie, cited in a helpful introduction to magical realism by Jackie Craven that informs some of my writing here (Craven 2019).
44 Magical realism originated from twentieth-century Latin America and nineteenth-century Russia "from colonised cultures, notably Alejo Carpentier, Jorge Luis Borges, Gabriel Garcia Marquez, Carlos Fuentes, Isabel Allende, and many more" (Bar-Am 2016) (page 387).
45 In every episode of the podcast, a different storyteller utilizes "high-sensory storytelling techniques to transport listeners to a time and place where everything changed for them" (https://meditativestory.com/).

46 This episode and its transcript URL are available here, and direct quotes are taken from it: https://meditativestory.com/david-whyte/.
47 Though the verbatim transcript is available online, this act helps me connect my senses (hearing) to the words on a page. Something happens within me as I hear the poet's voice, pause, see my hands turn his speech into a written discourse.
48 Most of the writing in this book is informed by my programme of research called Measuring Humanity, which "sought to co-produce a framework with marginalised community members and health practitioners that could systematically evaluate changes in 'softer' outcomes (such as trust) linked to health, wellbeing and inequalities. These aspects were to feed into more tangible 'harder' performance measures and targets saturating the health policy and practice landscape" (de Andrade 2018).
49 www.bbc.co.uk/history/historic_figures/blake_william.shtml (BBC History 2014).
50 Quotations come from a Meditative Story episode: https://meditativestory.com/david-whyte/.
51 These words are inspired by a pagan chant, "Round and Round We Dance." The origins of the chant could not be located, despite extensive online searches.
52 Despite its being well-known as a Pablo Picasso quote, searches for the conversation it originated from could not be located.

References

Ahmed, Sara. 2004. *The Cultural Politics of Emotion*. New York: Routledge.

Allen, Neil. 2009. "Is Capacity 'In Sight'?" *Journal of Mental Health Law* 168.

Antonovsky, Aaron. 1996. "The Salutogenic Model as a Theory to Guide Health Promotion." *Health Promotion International* 11 (1): 11–18.

Archer, Margaret, Roy Bhaskar, Andrew Collier, Tony Lawson, and Alan Norrie. 1998. "Critical Realism: Essential Readings." *Critical Realism: Essential Readings* (June): 1–756. https://doi.org/10.4324/9781315008592.

Bar-Am, Sonja. 2016. "First Episode Psychosis: A Magical Realist Guide Through Liminal Terrain." *Australian and New Zealand Journal of Family Therapy* 37 (3): 381–96. https://doi.org/10.1002/ANZF.1159.

Barnfield, Andrew. 2016. "Affect and Public Health – Choreographing Atmospheres of Movement and Participation." *Emotion, Space and Society* 20 (August): 1–9. https://doi.org/10.1016/J.EMOSPA.2016.04.003.

BBC History. 2014. "BBC – History – William Blake." *BBC*. www.bbc.co.uk/history/historic_figures/blake_william.shtml.

Cahnmann-Taylor, Melisa, and Richard Siegesmund. 2008. "Arts-Based Research in Education: Foundations for Practice." https://philpapers.org/rec/CAHARI.

Capra, Fritjof, and Pier Luigi Luisi. 2012. *The Systems View of Life: A Unifying Vision*. *The Systems View of Life*. Cambridge University Press. https://doi.org/10.1017/CBO9780511895555.

Chandler, Amy. 2012. "Self-Injury as Embodied Emotion Work: Managing Rationality, Emotions and Bodies." 46 (3): 442–57. https://doi.org/10.1177/0038038511422589.

Chandler, Amy, Rob Cover, and Scott J. Fitzpatrick. 2022. "Critical Suicide Studies, between Methodology and Ethics: Introduction." *Health (United Kingdom)* 26 (1): 3–9. https://doi.org/10.1177/13634593211061638.

Collins, Susan E. 2016. "Associations Between Socioeconomic Factors and Alcohol Outcomes." *Alcohol Research: Current Reviews* 38 (1): 83. /pmc/articles/PMC4872618/.

Cook, Christopher C. H. 2004. "Addiction and Spirituality." *Addiction (Abingdon, England)* 99 (5): 539–51. https://doi.org/10.1111/J.1360-0443.2004.00715.X.

Craven, Jackie. 2019. "Magical Realism – Definition and Examples." *ThoughtCo.* 2019. www.thoughtco.com/magical-realism-definition-and-examples-4153362.

Daykin, Norma, Karen Gray, Mel McCree, and Jane Willis. 2016. "Creative and Credible Evaluation for Arts, Health and Well-Being: Opportunities and Challenges of Co-Production." 9 (2): 123–38. https://doi.org/10.1080/17533015.2016.1206948.

de Andrade, Marisa de. 2017. "Validating The Feels – Measuring Humanity." *Measuring Humanity.* https://measuringhumanity.org/validating-the-feels.

———. 2018. "Measuring Humanity in Marginalised Communities – The Health Foundation." *The Health Foundation.* www.health.org.uk/blogs/measuring-humanity-in-marginalised-communities#:~:text=The project%2C now known as Measuring Humanity%2C sought,as trust%29 linked to health%2C wellbeing and inequalities.

de Andrade, Marisa de, and Nikolina Angelova. 2017. "An Asset-Based Indicator Framework: Using Co-Production, Co-Design and Innovative Methods to Engage with BME Groups." In *Glasgow Health and Social Care Partnership*, edited by G. Balint, B. Antala, C. Carty, J-M. A. Mabieme, I. B. Amar, and A. Kaplanova. https://doi.org/10.2/JQUERY.MIN.JS.

Driver, Michaela. 2010. "A 'Spiritual Turn' in Organizational Studies: Meaning Making or Meaningless?" 4 (1): 56–86. https://doi.org/10.1080/14766080709518646.

Felstiner Lowenthal, Mary. 1999. "Charlotte Salomon | Jewish Women's Archive." In *The Shalvi/Hyman Encyclopedia of Jewish Women.* https://jwa.org/encyclopedia/article/salomon-charlotte.

Foot, Jane. 2012. *What Makes Us Healthy?: The Asset Approach in Practice: Evidence, Action, Evaluation.* Asset Based Consulting. wmuh.pdf (assetbasedconsulting.co.uk)

Foster, Victoria. 2016. "Collaborative Arts-Based Research for Social Justice." In *Collaborative Arts-Based Research for Social Justice* (December): 63. https://doi.org/10.4324/9780203077450.

Frankl, Victor. 1984. *Man's Search for Meaning. Frontiers in Psychology.* New York. https://doi.org/10.3389/FPSYG.2016.01493.

Friedli, Lynne. 2013. "'What We've Tried, Hasn't Worked': The Politics of Assets Based Public Health 1." 23 (2): 131–45. https://doi.org/10.1080/09581596.2012.748882.

Friedli, Lynne, and Robert Stearn. 2015. "Positive Affect as Coercive Strategy: Conditionality, Activation and the Role of Psychology in UK Government Workfare Programmes." *Medical Humanities* 41 (1): 40–47. https://doi.org/10.1136/MEDHUM-2014-010622.

Hein, Serge F. 2018. "Deleuze, Immanence, and Immanent Writing in Qualitative Inquiry: Nonlinear Texts and Being a Traitor to Writing." 25 (1): 83–90. https://doi.org/10.1177/1077800418784328.

Holman Jones, Stacy, and Mark Pruyn. 2018. "Creative Selves/Creative Cultures: Critical Autoethnography, Performance, and Pedagogy." *Creative Selves/Creative Cultures* 11. https://doi.org/10.1007/978-3-319-47527-1_1.

Hustedde, Ronald J. 1998. "On the Soul of Community Development." *Journal of the Community Development Society* 29 (2): 153–65.

Jackson, Alecia, and Lisa a Mazzei. 2012. *Thinking with Theory in Qualitative Research: Viewing Data Across Multiple Perspectives. The Qualitative Report.* Vol. 20. New York: Routledge.

Katz, Amy S., Billie Jo Hardy, Michelle Firestone, Aisha Lofters, and Melody E. Morton-Ninomiya. 2019. "Vagueness, Power and Public Health: Use of 'Vulnerable' in Public Health Literature." 30 (5): 601–11. https://doi.org/10.1080/09581596.2019.1656800.

Law, John. 2004. *After Method: Mess in Social Science Research.* New York: Routledge.

Lewis, Aubrey. 1934. "The Psychopathology of Insight." *British Journal of Medical Psychology* 14 (4): 332. https://doi.org/10.1111/J.2044-8341.1934.TB01129.X.

Lowe, Toby, and Rob Wilson. 2017. "Playing the Game of Outcomes-Based Performance Management. Is Gamesmanship Inevitable? Evidence from Theory and Practice." *Social Policy & Administration* 51 (7): 981–1001. https://doi.org/10.1111/SPOL.12205.

Macintyre, Anna, Daniel Ferris, Briana Gonçalves, and Neil Quinn. 2018. "What Has Economics Got to Do with It? The Impact of Socioeconomic Factors on Mental Health and the Case for Collective Action." *Palgrave Communications* 4 (1): 1–5. https://doi.org/10.1057/s41599-018-0063-2.

McNiff, Shaun. 2008. "Art-Based Research." In *Handbook of the Arts in Qualitative Research: Perspectives, Methodologies, Examples, and Issues,* edited by J. G. Knowles, and A. L. Cole, 29–41. SAGE Publications, Inc. https://dx.doi.org/10.4135/9781452226545

Morgan, Jules. 2018. "The Hard Problem of Consciousness: Understanding Our Reality." Thousand Oaks, California. *The Lancet Neurology* 17 (5): 403. https://doi.org/10.1016/S1474-4422(18)30080-2.

Muir, John. 1911. *My First Summer in the Sierra. Sierra Club Books.* 1988th ed. Boston: Houghton Mifflin.

Office for Health Improvement and Disparities. 2013. *Public Health Outcomes Framework.* Government. www.gov.uk/government/collections/public-health-outcomes-framework.

Patel, Vikram, Shekhar Saxena, Crick Lund, Graham Thornicroft, Florence Baingana, Paul Bolton, Dan Chisholm, et al. 2018. "The Lancet Commission on Global Mental Health and Sustainable Development." *The Lancet* 392 (10157): 1553–98. https://doi.org/10.1016/S0140-6736(18)31612-X.

Rippon, Simon, and Trevor Hopkins. 2015. "Head, Hands and Heart: Asset-Based Approaches in Health Care – The Health Foundation." *The Health Foundation.* 2015. www.health.org.uk/publications/head-hands-and-heart-asset-based-approaches-in-health-care.

Ruth, Behar. 2008. "Between Poetry and Anthropology." In *Arts-Based Research in Education,* 63. New York: Routledge.

Scottish Community Development Centre. 2011. "Community Development and Co-Production: Issues for Policy and Practice." www.scdc.org.uk.

Sigerson, Debbie, and Laurence Gruer. 2011. *Asset-Based Approaches to Health Improvement.* Glasgow: NHS Health Scotland.

Smith, Katherine E., and Ted Schrecker. 2015. "Theorising Health Inequalities: Introduction to a Double Special Issue." *Social Theory and Health* 13 (3–4): 219–26. https://doi.org/10.1057/STH.2015.25.

Speedy, Jane. 2015. *Staring at the Park: A Poetic Autoethnographic Inquiry.* New York: Routledge.

Stearn, Robert, and Lynne Friedli. 2013. *Whistle While You Work (For Nothing): Positive Affect as Coercive Strategy – The Case of Workfare | Centre for Medical Humanities Blog.* Centre for Medical Humanities. https://medicalhumanities.wordpress.com/2013/12/10/whistle-while-you-work-for-nothing-positive-affect-as-coercive-strategy-the-case-of-workfare/#_edn1.

Tough, Hannah, Johannes Siegrist, and Christine Fekete. 2017. "Social Relationships, Mental Health and Wellbeing in Physical Disability: A Systematic Review." *BMC Public Health* 17 (1). https://doi.org/10.1186/S12889-017-4308-6.

Turner, Victor. 1967. *Betwixt-and-Between: The Liminal Period in Rites de Passage. In the Forest of Symbols: Aspects of Ndembu Ritual.* Ithaca, NY: Cornell University Press.

Tyler, Imogen. 2013. *Revolting Subjects: Social Abjection and Resistance in Neoliberal Britain,* 265. London: Zed Books.

White, Daniel. 2017. "Affect: An Introduction." *Cultural Anthropology* 32 (2): 175–80. https://doi.org/10.14506/CA32.2.01.

Wong, Paul, and Prem Fry. 1998. *The Human Quest for Meaning: A Handbook of Psychological Research and Clinical Applications.* Lawrence Erlbaum Associates Publishers. https://psycnet.apa.org/record/1998-06124-000.

2   Emergence – the gap between two epistemic bubbles

***

"Hello, Professor Ebba," I said with a wavering voice.

"Where are you?" She spoke quickly, without time for pleasantries.

I scanned my spellbinding surroundings, searching for the right words.

"I'm in the field," I eventually said.

"Get back," she barked. "Immediately. We've had a security breach."

A security breach? Impossible. Not with our firewalls and protocols.

"Professor Ebba, are you . . ."

"Get back immediately. Someone's hacked into The Walled Garden."

Blood drained from my head to my toes. The Walled Garden. It was worse than I had imagined.

SILLY's strict ethics and data protection protocols meant this shouldn't have happened. Couldn't have happened. This was The Institution's worst nightmare.

"Yes, Professor Ebba. Of course." The sun was rapidly disappearing into the bottom of the pear. Darkness was descending. The thought of leaving left me hollow. "Could it just be a glitch?"

"Get back immediately," she repeated. "The SANITY team is investigating as we speak. It's an extraordinary breach. Everything returned to normal within Planck Time . . ."

Tiny hairs stood up to attention on my arms. Planck Time, the smallest conceivable unit of time. A component to objectively measure cosmological forces that capture the essence of time flying by as if on its own life course or dragging its feet in the humdrum of life (Williams 2010).

"The breach was – or is – so subtle . . . almost imperceptible. . . . Every now and then a code changes. Then it changes back. Like a flicker. You see it, then it's gone," Ebba continued. "There's talk of some DPS going on."

"Data Packet Sniffing! I thought we were running an application to capture data packets?" My nontechy mind raced to make sense of this nonsensical development.

"We are. But if this is all true, it means technically someone can see your data."

I noticed at that moment how my core started convulsing, my extremities unexpectedly frozen.

DOI: 10.4324/9781003196488-2

In the periphery, I became aware of a blazing glow changing from an intense orange to bright white. With the help of eleven people, who had arrived out of nowhere, Sara had started a bonfire. One by one, they threw broken branches into a bottomless pit. This, the full moon and the stars, and some solar lights scattered around The Futile Forest were our only light. The night had well and truly replaced a day riddled with uncertainties.

"Get back immediately," Professor Ebba repeated. "And be careful." She hung up.

I sat there for what felt like an eternity, wrapping my arms around myself, blowing cold air into my hands.

Too much information to process.

Too short a space of time.

We're such badly built machines, I caught myself thinking.
  We humans.

  We think we're so smart and sophisticated, but we're full of flaws. Layer
upon layer
    upon layer
  of unprocessed thoughts and memories and nightmares.
    And dreams.
    All just accumulating.   Amounting to nothing.

By now, Sara stood at my side, watching me tremble, warming me once again from the inside out. She said nothing, just stood there in all her power.

"What are you going to do?" she finally asked, her left arm gesturing to a circle of humans that had formed around the flames, trancelike.

I looked beyond her fingertips. Nothing but black skies and a ball of fire.
I thought about what I should have been doing.
Escaping.
Working within the walls of institutional safeguards and protocols. But I couldn't shift it, that feeling.

I'm almost there,

I reminded myself.

Just need some more time and context to piece it altogether,

I reminded myself.

I ignored the wave of nausea crashing at my throat.

As a hypnotic drumbeat emerged from the circular gathering, I found myself serenely drifting towards these strangers who held some secret to a mindset that was still a mystery to me. A mystery to others. The mystery of madness. I joined them in orbit as if I had no say in the matter. As if I was surrendering to the possibility of peace for just one day. There was something magical about the moment.

That magic was my reality.

***

INTERLUDE – (MAGICAL, EVIDENCE-BASED) REALITY AND THE HUMAN CONDITION

Reader, what are you reading right now?

Almost certainly, you'll conceive of this tale as a story – a narrative, a written text – though hopefully evoking some moving images and noises in the movie and soundtrack of your mind.

You'll have noted an "irreducible element of magic" alongside a "strong presence of the phenomenal world" (Faris 2004).[1] This magic is very much taken for granted in Sara's world in The Futile Forest. This magic is Sara's reality.

Perhaps this makes you feel a little uneasy, particularly in a text claiming to be methodologically suitable for public health. You may "experience some unsettling doubts" as you try "to reconcile two contradictory understanding of events," especially as the narrative "merges different realms" and "disturbs received ideas about time, space, and identity" (Faris 2004).[2]

Maybe you're wondering, "Is the magic understood as supernatural, or merely a way of looking at reality? Is the magic inherent in reality or is it purely textual?" (Aldea 2011).[3]

To this I say, exorcise yourself. Banish, for the duration of this book at least, the belief system that's a particular kind of knowing that will get you to the other side of knowledge.

Trust in the process of reading, writing, and researching that will allow you to hear (at the very least) *two* competing voices. One that is clearly logical, rational, and realistic. Another one that simply believes in magic (Spindler 1993).

For this to work, you'll need to (as I have) accept the inherent inconsistency between the two paradigms and go with the collective unconscious of Sara's reality in The Futile Forest. You'll have to accept the worldviews of the other Community Members that the anonymous researcher and you are about to meet.

Not only is this metaphysical magical realism valid and real for those who're living, breathing, and trying to communicate it, but their so-called alternative reality is also borne from necessity. Sara and her fellow Community Members are marginalised – or colonised – "others" trying, and quite often failing, to find their identity in a place that rejects their beliefs as equivalent to science, the biomedical model, and Western rationality.[4]

They believe in the power of their own magic. Their magic is healing. The problem is that others – health professionals and other agencies and services – don't. They think their magic is madness.

So where do we go from here?

I'm drawn to a key health humanities[5] text that cites shamanism alongside studies in transcultural psychiatry exploring dissociative experiences – "typically sudden, time-limited alterations in identity, behaviour and mental state."[6] I wonder what their identity was to begin with. And who defined them as such at "baseline" then "measured" their mental state as it altered along a trajectory of trance, dance, soul retrieval, and ritualistic movement. How did the researcher know their shamanic journeys involved a drifting into detachment from reality? What was real to begin with? And what was the assumption about our reality that was being taken for granted in that study?

Intrigued, I dig out the original publication in *Journal of Trauma & Dissociation*. Its aim is "to determine whether classical culture-bound syndromes occur among [100] psychiatric inpatients with dissociative disorders in North America." Means of data collection and measurement scales include "the Dissociative Trance Disorder Interview Schedule, the Dissociative Experiences Scale (DES), and the Dissociative Disorders Interview Schedule." This is a solid research design with scientific objectivity and reliability in mind, clearly seeking to eliminate bias (Ross, Schroeder, and Ness 2013).[7]

I learn that the DES is the most popular self-report measure of dissociation and is as statistically sound as it gets. After analysis, you're left with respondents in two groups: "those with pathological dissociative experiences (in the dissociative taxon) and those without."[8]

I'm both impressed and troubled. Does this mean someone is "in" or "out" of what is deemed to be a "normal" and appropriate range of experiencing reality by self-reporting on their experience of reality? I guess the "test-retest reliability" measure is meant to check-recheck that they were firmly grounded in reality – or not – when they first completed then recompleted the test?

But how can we be certain that the psychiatric inpatients weren't being contacted by spiritual ancestors while being tested?

What if they called on the spirits to help them convince the researchers that they were absolutely fine, that they fall within a completely "normal spectrum of reality," to allow the inpatients to continue to do their work as healers? To help them help others tap into spiritual practices to find inner peace and begin to change the troubled world we live in?

However convoluted this thesis may sound, perhaps it needs to be taken as seriously as any other argument when the starting point for analysis is an accepted – albeit "altered" – state of reality.

What is clear is that "we" – largely Western scholars designing studies informed by the dominant scientific paradigm – have a pathologised, taken-for-granted definition of what is and is not an acceptable version of reality that sets the stage for what follows in diagnosis, management, treatment, and acceptability.

This helps us put inpatients (or outpatients, or Community Members) and their illnesses in a very particular place – for their benefit as much as ours – as this is a system that standardises data to help us reach firm conclusions and make solid recommendations to improve health.

In this paper, the data on "possession states and related experiences" can be used to monitor and regulate "behavioural dyscontrol, shouting, echolalia [repeating words or sounds that don't appear to make sense], confusion, crying, exaggerated startle, and, in the case of amok, attempts to kill others, which may be successful" (Ross, Schroeder, and Ness 2013).[9]

I'd never given "amok" much thought, but reading it in this culturally bound context makes me feel uneasy. I learn through a quick check with *Merriam-Webster* that the official definition is,

> An episode of sudden mass assault against people or objects usually by a single individual following a period of brooding that has traditionally been regarded as occurring especially in Malaysian culture but is now increasingly viewed as psychopathological behaviour occurring worldwide in numerous countries and cultures.
>
> (Merriam-Webster 2022)

The notion that *one* unacceptable "psychopathological" behavioural state, as described in the *Diagnostic and Statistical Manual of Mental Disorders (DSM) – IV*, published by the *American* Psychiatric Association, is *Malaysian* while another "pibloktoq is limited to *Arctic Inuit* populations," while another "ataque de nervios occurs primarily in *Puerto Rico*," stirs up more discomfort within me (Ross, Schroeder, and Ness 2013).[10]

It suggests to me, perhaps implicitly, that madness is attributed to other cultures – non-Western ones – that deviate from the norm.

This may imply that other cultures aren't safe enough or can't be trusted.

Perhaps it subconsciously plants a seed that I should be on the lookout if or when I come into contact with someone who may look or sound a little (or very) different to me, as they could be about to say or do something that isn't quite right or even potentially dangerous.

This may mean I find myself choosing another seat on the bus. Or reporting a suspicious-looking person because I suspect they're repeatedly muttering something under their breath (that I can't understand) or they simply have a strange look in their eyes.

These thoughts make me feel uncomfortable. Living in a world like this makes me feel uneasy. I'm left slightly on edge. The more I read about people like this doing things like that on my social media feeds or see them having "episodes" on the twenty-four-hour rolling news agenda – the same words and headlines and images over and over and over again – the more I feel stressed out about this.

I find my heart racing a little when the "DUN DUNN DUNN DINNNNGGGG" news jingle at the top of the hour reminds me that we're in trouble. That I'm in trouble. I'm starting to feel stressed out about this, maybe even a tad paranoid. When I leave the house to buy milk at my corner shop, I see someone who could be them, who might be thinking of doing something like that. My fists clench. My mind races. I must get out of here. I run the three blocks back in a state, shut the door behind me, lean against the door, and remind myself that no one can get me here. No one at all.

I have no family around me. I'm single. My friends are busy. I'm okay here. I'm safe here. Alone, behind closed doors. Day in and day out.

On day 63 of this pattern, I go to my doctor to get some help. I think I'm depressed. I think something's wrong with me, I tell them.

Help me. Somebody help me.

I'm given some antidepressants and put on the eight-week waiting list for talking therapy.

I wait. And wait and wait.

Meanwhile, I watch the news, over and over again.

It's an uncomfortable ending for me as I eat and drink myself into oblivion.

Until someone finds me cold.[11]

Deep breath.

Somewhere out there, there's an alternative story playing out in a cosy, pre-Covid therapy room where – and when – feeling soft furnishings and holding hardbacks were permissible. There – here – you're not a client, you're a person, with a cotton-wool blanket wrapped around you as you sink into an armchair that holds you while the therapist in front of you holds the space.

It's an oddly intimate affair for two strangers, especially as you're meant to tell them your deepest, darkest secrets and trust that the professional code of ethics they're bound by is watertight.

There's also something slightly suspicious about starting a pact with this person in front of you, who looks nice enough with their neatly pressed navy shirt and soft and slightly sleepy eyes but, let's not forget, is a stranger. A complete stranger. One with credentials in person-centred care or psychodynamic theory or some other variation of counselling and/or psychotherapy, but still as unspecified as a stoic voice in a confessional box.

Still, you enter into a silent agreement. You tell them your secrets. They hear you with nonjudgemental awareness. You both see what unfolds.

The setting is more than a little mad, you deduce, but you go along with it and decide to play by their rules for a few sessions, just to see where this may take you. You're appeasing them really. Accepting their evidently distorted version of reality for an hour at a time – well, for fifty minutes – what's known as the counselling hour. They even make up their own timekeeping system.

Somewhere along the way, maybe during your fourth or fifth week, something magical happens. You're finding it difficult to put into words, but you know it happened because you were there and you know it to be real and true.

You were sharing something intimate with this now-not-so-new-stranger. You'd become accustomed to the smell of their orange-blossom diffuser. Their long pauses no longer felt disinterested or agonising, but rather reflective. As if someone was listening to you – as if someone could hear you – for the very first time in your life. Right there, in that holding space, you experience a state of altered consciousness.

This has happened to "Eva" – an anonymised "client" in Sonja Bar-Am's (Bar-Am 2016) paper that hears and makes meaning of Eva's first episode of psychosis through a liminal landscape of magical realism.

I came across this paper when pulling together my proposal for this book in the middle of the night, eleven months ago now.[12]

At that time, I had the bare bones of an idea for a creative (non)fiction text proposing post-qualitative methodological approaches to a public health audience. I wanted the book to begin midbreakthrough as the author, a public health policy researcher, woke up in a vaporous, altered state of mind, body, and soul.

In my mind, she was literally wedged between two paradigms – (i) Public Health and (ii) Health Humanities and Arts – that had taken the form of soapy, knowledge bubbles.

My character's first preoccupation, in her then formless state, was to make sense of her new identity. She knew she wasn't real, but what was she?

Suspended between these seemingly oppositional standpoints – and longing to be grounded – she turned to the scientific literature's understanding of realism, truth, representativeness, materiality, and corporeality alongside "other" interpretations of these concepts to see if there were overlaps in the humanities and arts.

It struck her (well, me) that the two fields she was crisscrossing, and therefore her very existence, have very different beliefs about "what is real and what is not."

I imagined her typing these words into an internet search. I did the same thing.

The word *psychosis* appeared.

This, I realised, was an important place to start her (my) journey of unpacking reality through magical realism.

Psychosis. A loaded construct that pathologises the human condition. A medical label that is, at its core, about a person's experience of reality, ironically diagnosed through language based on the subjective view (albeit based on "objective criteria") of an expert who clearly lives in a different (evidence-based) reality from the person being assessed.

A deep dive into the academic literature threw up just two papers engaging directly with psychosis and magical realism in health settings, though none specifically in public health. Bar-Am's seminal paper in her field was the first I encountered. Positioned in counselling and psychotherapy, it explored narratives of psychotic episodes and proposed that "a magical realist listening position supports a non-pathologising, helpful, and meaningful exploration of psychotic content (hearing voices, hallucinations, thoughts, rituals)," and that "therapists may be aided by mapping a client's narrated content along the separation, liminal and convergence phases of a rite of passage metaphor" (Bar-Am 2016).[13]

The research engaged with words like *rhizome* (a concept I'd become familiar with in discussions with colleagues who are themselves counsellors or psychotherapists). I knew words like *affect* and *assemblages* were likely to appear too – there's an entire body of literature waiting to be explored that public health researchers may have encountered at some point in their undergraduate or postgraduate degrees but tend not to engage with in their discipline or day-to-day work.

I wanted my character to fill this gap, invigorating conventional approaches to public health. I wanted her to pour post-qualitative methodological insights with firm, philosophical reflections into the public health canon so studies designed in this way would be both creative and credible.

I wanted her to respectfully acknowledge books engaging with public health methodologies that are largely situated in positivist, quantitative paradigms suggesting that the "essential" research methods in the field should be shaped by predictability, objectivity, generalisability, and validity. She would also give a nod to qualitative paradigms though notice that they are often bundled under the banner of "interpretivism."

With an odd exception, my character would notice that there is limited engagement with ontology and epistemology in public health, as reality and knowledge in these texts tend to be grounded in scientific assumptions that do not require further consideration or justification.

Public health books that engage with qualitative or creative methods (usually positioned as community engagement or participatory action research) only scratch the surface of the possibilities that arts-based theories and methodologies can bring to the discipline. I wanted my character to "validate the feels," to challenge traditional public health assumptions by situating the reader in alternative realities where knowledge, evidence, data collection, and analysis take on new meanings for participants and researchers.

But rather than telling – which is what most public health books tend to do, either by instructing academics "how to do" research in a particular way or telling them how this research has been conducted through examples or case studies – I wanted her *to show* readers alternative theories and methods *by doing*.

In my mind, the learning would be embedded within a creative product, which in itself would be evidence of the methodology in action. The result would be a metaphysical creation that endeavoured to be both educational and entertaining.

While the "real worlds" in the stories portrayed would have an obvious tinge of magic or fantasy, they would be grounded in the "real world," substantiated by the academic literature, and informed by findings from multiple datasets in my Measuring Humanity research programme. This would further trouble public health's attachment to objective reality in evidence gathering.

This all seemed imminently possible when I came across "Eva's" story, told so eloquently by (or rather *with*) her academic narrator, Sonja (I feel like we should be on first-name terms), who describes herself "as a family and relationship counsellor practicing narrative therapy with its backdrop of post-structuralism and curiosity of exploring new entry points for narratives of identity" (Bar-Am 2016).[14]

There's a lot going on in that title, but perhaps the take-home messages for me would be a focus on the relational and the power embedded in discourse (conversations, exchanges, counselling, storytelling, publishing). The push against post-positivism and belief that an absolute truth can ever be found, while using critical theory to push for change. And that it is through the practice of telling-writing-saying-expressing-hearing that meanings, relations, and identities are interpreted.

Without speaking for her or making assumptions, Sonja's work would be to sit with "Eva" (I'm going to drop the quotation marks from now on; I assume you know by now that Eva is both real and unreal) to make sense of her reality *with her*. A process that entails "a rhizomic-like convergence of the real and the magical in listening to [Eva's] experiences of reality moving through a psychosis" (Bar-Am 2016).[15]

I first encountered *rhizome* in this context when I stumbled upon a translation of Deleuze (the French philosopher) and Guattari's (the French psychoanalyst and political activist) *Anti-Oedipus* (Deleuze and Guattari 2000). It was cited in a Counselling Studies postgraduate student's thesis and left me a little dizzy. Gilles and Félix, respectively, offered an affirmative account of schizophrenia so enigmatic when compared to the ones I'd come across in public health publications.

One way to explain it would be to note that "the schizophrenic's expressions seem incoherent and confused to us . . . because he does not use the organization and representations of common sense" in the way in which we might expect them to. But this doesn't mean the schizophrenic is delusional or hallucinating, but rather that they aren't subscribing to our very rigid representations of reality that only permit particular possibilities: "in representing something, one can recognize a conceptual identity, an analogy of judgement, a similarity in perception or an opposition to something imagined; through representation one can thus only think identity, analogy, similarity and opposition" (Deleuze and Guattari 2000).[16]

It's liberating to blow open the possibility of something that isn't "this" as opposed to "that." "Good" as opposed to "bad." "Normal" as opposed to "abnormal." Just a spectrum of experiences that spread out like plants with roots and shoots and spurts that go whichever which way they please rather than following linear, treelike trajectories. Just like rhizomes.

Back in the counselling room, Eva speaks while Sonja listens, and their rhizomatic dialogue goes places. It spreads out to fill magical, liminal spaces – "an idea of nomadic thought and nomadic identity through a psychotic episode" emerges (Bar-Am 2016).[17]

Sonja invites Eva to "think of it as the psychosis taking [her] on a journey through some new landscape of [her] mind" (Bar-Am 2016).[18] As I understand it, Eva (with Sonja) uses magical realism to make sense of her identity, much like I am using magical realism to make sense of (evidence-based) reality as conceptualised and applied in public health.

Pause.

I realise, reader, this stream of consciousness outpour started in that orange-blossomed counselling room, where I first told you about an experience of a state of altered consciousness in a therapeutic session.

What I haven't told you yet is that there are words for these intimate moments in the psychotherapy literature, even though words don't come close to explaining what happens behind closed doors when this moment happens – "when I am somehow in touch with the unknown in me, when perhaps I am in a slightly altered state of consciousness in the relationship, then whatever I do seems to be full of healing," when I am "part of something larger. Profound growth and heal-ing and energy are present" (Sanders, Frankland, and Wilkins 2009).[19]

When you are relating so deeply that you feel alive, awake. When you experience reality as something different. When you feel much lighter, clearer. Lucid. When you experience an alternative perception of time (Mearns and Cooper 2005).

I think about Wendy Faris's words as I drift back to The Futile Forest: "[the] magical realist narrative resembles the performance of a shaman who constructs a persona and a discourse that imaginatively negotiate different realms, joining the everyday world of concrete reality and the world of the spirits" (Faris 2004).[20]

***

Gong. Gooooonnnnnnnngggggg.

The drumming stopped, and another sound emerged. A humming.

"Sat Nam, Sat Nam, Sat Nam, Sat Nam . . ."

What are they saying? I wondered.

"I am truth. Truth is my essence. Truth is my identity," Sara whispered. She stood at my side like a light in the dark, her pencil arms glow sticks in the night.

Who is this human who can read my mind? I wondered.

No response from Sara or the one, two, eleven . . . twenty-four, fifty . . . sixty-four humans who were part of the circle I was in.

Where had they appeared from?

Sixty-four humans in a semicomatose state, seemingly unaffected by the unmistakable sound of a gong in the sky. Not the clanging kind that attaches to your nerve endings and induces bloodcurdling shrieks in your head as your inner voice tries to get it to quieten down. More the type that bathes you in almond milk infused with manuka honey and camomile.

Good for the mind, good for the body.

"Why aren't they moving?" I whispered back. "They look suspiciously dead on their feet."

Their eyes closed, their feet hip distance apart, their bodies open, their palms facing outward, their heads tipped upwards the blue. All sixty-four of them, spread evenly 'round a black-box sphere that seemed to have two secretive entrances that also served as exits.

"They're preparing for their journeys. In a moment, there'll be a window of insight.[21] A window of light."

"What are you . . . ?"

"Watch this."

The concrete walls, only seconds before black blank canvasses, metamor-phosed into 4DX banners. A glorious corona (a circle of light, not a virus) spread concentrated doses of vitamin D so real you wouldn't believe you weren't being warmed by the real thing.

"Five minutes of this top-up and they're set for the day. Or night. Just the right amount of energy to get them through up to twenty hours of darkness. We've figured out the algorithm," Sara explained.

I watched as life swiftly seeped into sixty-four specimens. A softening began.

"How often does this happen?" I asked, melting with them.

"Every day. Every day before the Hour of Sharing and Stillness."

It was quite the vision to behold.

"Follow the sun," Sara exhaled, her eyes still closed.

"What are you . . . ?" I asked quietly, my eyes wide open, trying to take it all in.

"Follow the sun. That's [Rule # 2]. Spacetimemattering."[22]

She said it as if it were one word. No spaces, no hyphens, just three words stuck together after an instruction that would have sounded surreal if we'd been in the tropics but seemed insane in this black, concrete green space suspended in the skies, perched over a damp and disadvantaged neighbourhood that hardly ever saw sunshine.

Years and years of studying and researching health and never had I ever come across this concept. It had to be made up.

"It's a real thing. Trust me." Sara's words resonated with a second, prolonged *goooooonnnng*.

As the sound bounced off the sides of the high-est-rise building, I sensed, only for a second, that I was tapping into some sort of mental state – not quite conscious, not quite unconscious, but sort of sitting somewhere in between. Sensing something – parts of me, parts of "them" maybe. Sensing something I wasn't quite fully aware of yet. It was just outside the reach of my mind, but it was there. I could feel it.[23]

At once, there was movement in complete silence. The bodies shuffled round the boundaries of their circle, some moving a bit closer to the glowing embers in the centre to warm their hands, others seating themselves on the solid ground. They all seemed at home, as if they knew what was coming next.

"Come with me."

Sara, whose strides had become more regal, led me to a space in the circle with a throne-cum-half-bed-cum-cushioned-cathedra. "Take a seat," she gestured. "That shawl is for you. I thought you might get a bit chilly."

It took me a moment to realise I was actually shivering. I reached for the thin stole, which was the colour of sunshine. It was made of the same fabric as Sara's delicate purple one, still draped at her elbows, but deceptively warm and soft. Shakes of electricity pushed through me as the scarf touched my skin, creating a circuit of comfort.

Sara's cheeks glowed, even in the darkness.

"We used to make our way into the circle two by two, coming in from those opposite access points." She pointed to a couple of black holes in the distance. "One of us would walk this way and grab a grey blanket, the other that way and get a red one. Grey, red, grey, red. We'd walk down the dividing aisle draped in our blankets and split to our sides, where we'd settle on our numbered spots on the ground."

I followed her finger. M1, B1, M2, B2, M3, B3 . . . *all the way to M32, B32.*
MIND-BODY BOUNDARY, PLEASE DO NOT CROSS OVER YOUR

RESPECTIVE DIVISION was barely distinguishable in what looked like white chalk on the brickwork.

"Then one day something shifted. We realised we could make our own choices, we were free to be who we wanted to be, so we started taking whichever blanket appealed to us that day and sat wherever we felt like in the circle. Life made a lot more sense. It all became much more chilled."

I looked at the shapeless grey-red forms in the night. They looked rather relaxed to me.

"I'm not sure I'm following the logic here. What's with the dividing line? And why would you all be walking this middle path anyway?"

I tried to take in the sixty-four people surrounding me, half in red, half in grey, all in darkness. They'd stopped their small talk; 128 eyes were firmly fixed on me.

"Well, that depends on how we were diagnosed. With problems of the mind. Or problems of the body," a thin voice chimed from the dark, "as if that's how it works."

The others nodded and muttered in agreement.

"We knew something was up. Something serious. They were after us. Trying to take away our freedom, trying to tell us what was wrong with us, getting it so completely wrong. Taking us away from ourselves, away from the people we loved, away from each other. Locking us up. If not real prison, then mind prison. We had to do something. We had to put our heads, hearts, and bodies together," the same tinny tone disclosed, though her voice seemed to be getting louder. Stronger.

"And one day, it all made sense." A giant shadow appeared on the 4DX banners pretending to be the sun. Like a phoenix rising from the ashes, the silhouette grew bigger and bigger until it shape-shifted to become a small human.[24]

"That's Mary," Sara whispered as the figure settled into an emerald-coloured sling made of fabric, a solid rope and some netting suspended between two hardwood trees that had anchored themselves in the middle of the circle.

"What's she lying on?" I was transfixed as Mary closed her eyes and spread herself out corpse-like, her body held by this material container that hadn't existed only moments before.

"The Hammock of Happiness."

     Doom.

          Doom.

          Da-doom.

"It's where the healing happens."

                    Doom.

Doom.

          Doom.

"As soon as we found SANITY," Mary continued as she lay there looking asleep, "it all made sense."

          Da-doom.

                Doom.

"Did she say you all found SANITY?" I turned to Sara, whose eyes were also now shut as she held a goatskin handheld drum in her left hand and a repurposed branch with a padded, match-like end.

My mind was trying to make sense of all this, and I was struggling. Really struggling. How could The Community have created SANITY? Security Analysis and Network Information Technology was the brainchild of The Institution. I was certain of it. Professor Ebba's call still rang in my ears, alongside the sound of drumming. Soft. Softer still. Sturdier. Stronger. Loud. Louder. Seven, eleven, twenty-seven. Sixty-four drumbeats sounding in unison.

"Get back immediately," I heard Professor Ebba shout in my mind. *"The SANITY team is investigating as we speak. It's an extraordinary breach. Everything returned to normal within Planck Time . . ."*

"Yes," Sara replied. "We all found SANITY."

Soar so tall

Spinning the cosmos

on wings of sheer fire

Hey fly o free o

o free o free o

Hey fly o free o

o free o free o

"Soar like a phoenix
Soar like a phoenix

Soar so tall

Spinning the cosmos

on wings of sheer fire

Hey fly o free o

o free o free o

Hey fly o free o

o free o free o."[25]

Sweet chanting. Call and respond. As if both sides were hearing each other so clearly and celebrating their oneness. Over and over and over again as Mary lay there in a hammock, looking so serene, as a ripple of rhythm transported us elsewhere. Next to her, a tiny statue of a pine marten had emerged, moulded from clay.

Someone stepped out, almost as if they were being carried by the beat rather than their own feet. With their eyes closed, they glided to Mary and placed trembling hands on her slight shoulders.

"That's Lucy," Sara mouthed, as this Community Member moved one palm to Mary's forehead and another to the base of her neck. She wore an oversized baby-pink crystal around her neck, suspended from a thick silver chain that also carried a cross. Ginger curls framed her flushed, focused face.

It looked as if her shut eyelids were staring at something in the distance, something silent that was telling her something, something that was channelling something. I followed what would have been her gaze if she'd actually been looking at something, but saw nothing bar a thick plume of smoke coming from non-existent incense sticks.

A warm ray of sunshine cut through a massive sheet of glass and rested on Mary's essence. We were no longer at the top of a concrete building but surrounded by some body of water. A lake perhaps, with little waves lapping at our feet. The air smelt of sweet rose and pine.

"Swirl and swirl together
> our fingers weaved together.
Swirl and swirl together
> our fingers weaved together.
Breathing our being in a sphere of love.
> Our connection is deep and the swirl continues."[26]

The drumming continued as another Community Member stepped in from the circle and placed his hands on Mary's feet. Her body jolted as if she'd been plugged in to a live socket. He responded with an involuntary shake.

There was something truly special about this person. I found myself sinking deeper into my body, taking fuller breaths and feeling warmed by an imaginary electric blanket he seemed to be carrying. I could imagine him walking on the water encompassing us.

Mary's body took one last quiver as he lifted his thin fingers from her ankles and placed them on a bronze singing bowl sitting beneath the hammock on a woven cushion. A final shiver rushed through him to his fingertips as he lifted the bowl into the light and orbited it with a baton. As vibrations reverberated, the drumming began to subside.

He was on one knee, with his right arm reaching to the sky, with bowl in his hand, as if proposing to the sky. Then on both knees, he reached for a flute, and with a few silky tootle-toos, he gently brought the circle to a close.

A safe silence for what felt like eternity, then deep breaths all 'round as we all arrived back in The Futile Forest from wherever we'd just been. Everyone was smiling.

"Connected. Let's never forget that we're all connected in mind, body, and soul. And the world out there" – Sara pointed to the edge of the building – "isn't real. This is. Don't ever get lost in the illusion of life. Remember at all times that this is our reality."

The Community Members nodded or sat still in quiet assurance.

"Would anyone like to share anything?" Sara prompted.

"Only that I owe my life to you all," someone said. They were dressed in jeans and a dirty white T-shirt. "Only yesterday I was standing on the high street in the rain, opposite the off-license, thinking about the bottle of vodka I wanted to have in my hand, and then I remembered. This, this street with these people looking at me sideways as if I don't matter, these people who don't really see me . . ."

"We've got you, sister," Sara said as tears arrived.

"I feel sorry for them," the Community Member continued. "They don't know what I know. They don't know what we know. They call me crazy 'cos they just don't get it."

"Aho, sister!" Sara bellowed.

"AHO!" came a chorus of greetings.

Sara must have noticed the look on my face.

"It's Native American. It means we're all related."

"But we're in Beguile," I reminded her, "nowhere near the Americas."

"We're all related." She smiled knowingly, as if she was the carrier of some best-kept secret. I look around at all the lit-up faces and saw the same look spread across them too.

How to describe what I could see between their relaxed brows and gentle expressions? How could this Community of mentally ill people present as so calm, non-threatening, insightful, certain?

"I just don't know what's going on here," I eventually conceded to them all. "Did Mary say you all found SANITY?"

"Yes," came the confident refrain from The Community.

"You've created Security Analysis and Network Information Technology?" I sounded meek.

"No," came their collective response.

"The Institution created that," Sara confirmed. "As you know." There wasn't a drop of animosity in her voice. I was none the wiser.

"We found sanity in each other," she said.

"We found sanity by coming together," Mary added.

"We found sanity by trying to make sense of The Institution's SANITY," a third voice added. It came from the opposite side of the circle. It belonged to Lucy. "Do you know what they're doing to us?"

"To you?" I asked.

"To all of us, but especially us." She gestured to the Community Members gathered around her on top of a building touching the sky.

I thought about what she was asking, tried to make sense of her question. A question that somehow had me caught up in the middle of it as a researcher at The Institution.

"No, I don't," I admitted. "I actually don't know what you're talking about. And you know what else? There's a big part of me that just wants to go home right now." I was thinking about the curried lentil soup in my stocked fridge and my warm living room that I could boost to even toastier settings from an app called Smarter on my phone. I was thinking that in a matter of moments (as soon as I figured out how to leave this alternative reality), I could be back to my domestic comforts, far removed from all The Community's . . . what was this anyway? Distress? Trauma? I didn't want to be there anymore; I wanted to escape.

"I know it's a lot to take in," Sara said steadily, "and the easiest thing to do is to run away. Run away from the truth, run away from reality." They were all nodding again. "But we're here to tell you that it doesn't have to be that way. Let me take you back to a moment in time that might be helpful."

The sensor-synchronised 4DX screens surrounding them that had just been the sun became something else. A replica of Sara popped out in all four dimensions. The real Sara and I, along with all the Community Members present, were watching her lying on a couch, or something that looked like a couch.

Sara was in a room – a clinical setting. There was someone else there, someone who looked distinctly familiar. I could hear Sara's thoughts as she spoke to this other person in her mind.

I remember the day my head went pop as if it were today, this moody Monday. Surrounded by memory foam, I sank into the spongy cocoon and settled as my mind metamorphosised. Blinked into the next-generation device in my palm, as a smile slid across my lips.

"Was it scary? No, not for me. Quite the contrary." We watched as Sara uncrossed her legs. Collapsed onto the black cushioned couch.

As if the tiny valve implanted in my head took the decision to release three decades of pressure, of analysing and organising, of thoughts, of memories, of feelings and patterns, of places, of faces of people, of smells. Of reality.

"What is reality? Nine-tenths of perception, I guess."

I tried, then stopped trying, to push against the flood that drenched my neurotransmitters and stopped them from sparking. Electrocuted, I stared at the screen that repeated the same words and images that just the day before had been cryptic clues and egoic displays of distorted selves on virtual platforms that stole and constructed people's identities simultaneously.

Everyone was suddenly bare, but they couldn't see their pointy nipples or flabby bum cheeks or citrus-peel thighs the colour of burnt figs. They were too busy making fruitless conversation and being aubergine, the colour of the season. Fake tans to go with bogus bylines and cringeworthy captions in make-believe worlds. Smiling as if their lives depended on it. Smiling in spite of their lives. In spite of life. As I know it.

"HALLELUJAH!" I wanted to screech from between the bedsheets as I watched the spectacle unfold, felt the fog finally lifting for the first time. Little droplets once sliding into puddles in the sky became suspended in a momentary haze, then evaporated.

"Euphoric relief."

An elaborate hoax.

If only someone had warned me that once I could see that the Emperor was naked, I would never be able to unsee his privates. I didn't ask for this discerning, twenty-twenty vision. There's a reason your body holds what your brain wants to forget. A reason for drugs in a class of their own, brews that blow your mind, talent contests that melt the minutes away.

"Sara, when was the last time this happened?"

The scene kept playing on the 4DX screens, but I could no longer follow it. I recognised that voice.

Sara was unmistakeably speaking to Professor Ebba.

***

INTERLUDE – TRAUMA TAKES CENTRE STAGE

Too far-fetched? How much of this scene are you willing to accept as real or discard as fabrication?

To be fully on board as a reader – and writer – of magical realist fiction, you

> must look beyond the realistic detail and accept the dual ontological structure of the text, in which the natural and the supernatural, the explainable and the miraculous, coexist side by side in a kaleidoscopic reality, whose apparently random angles are deliberately left to the audience's discretion.
>
> (Arva 2008).[27]

Perhaps you can see the value of this in a novel that, on the surface of it, was created to entertain like Haruki Murakami's *Kafka on the Shore*, where one character is a tracker of lost cats in a world where cats talk to people and fish fall from the sky.

Dig a little deeper, though, and even this creative product becomes a blank sheet for psychoanalytic theory, embodiment, healing, and symbolic order to be applied and explored. Seminal thinkers in liminality, post-structuralism, postmodern philosophy, and psychoanalysis have proposed contradictory interpretations of Murakami's novel – and even his publisher played with the multiple meanings of the book by inviting readers to make sense of it.[28]

Let's pause for a moment to muse on what scholarly sense-making may emerge from this novel using what Counsellor and Psychotherapist Nini Fang calls "imaginal dialogue as method of narrative inquiry." This is the method she used to describe her own pretend conversation with Virginia Woolf to epitomise the potential of reading as an "embodied, co-constructed interplay between the reader and the text" (Fang 2020).[29]

In fact, let's go one step further and put imaginal dialogue *to work* using the creative-relational approach this scholar writes about.

Here's an excerpt from an exchange I had with Nini and some other authors and thinkers. Well, I didn't actually talk to them – I'm making this dialogue up drawing from my imagination, Nini's paper, some carefully selected quotes from literary (magical realism) theorists, and a few novelists renowned for magical realism.[30]

NINI FANG: *"I came to explore the method of imaginal dialogue in response to the question of narratability of trauma. How do we narrate trauma, when the intensity of emotional registers disrupted the ordinary capacity to make sense of the experience?"* (Fang 2020).[31]

MARISA: I'm not entirely sure yet. This is something I'm trying to do in this book, too, using magical realism as a mechanism. I wonder if Nakata might know. The character portrayed as the elderly gent who talks to cats in *Kafka on the Shore*? Doesn't he carry the collective, intergenerational trauma of Japanese military history on his slight shoulders? The flashbacks of the Second World War? The fear of attack – real or imagined? Small wonder he ends up collapsed and unconscious in some forest. Small wonder he can't remember much and has somehow forgotten how to read. Talk about wiping the trauma slate clean.

MURAKAMI: Yes. *"Memories warm you up from the inside. But they also tear you apart"* (Murakami 2005).

MARISA: So we should try to forget those memories that have caused us too much pain? Push them out of our minds and bodies and souls entirely so they can't frighten us anymore?

MURAKAMI: Hmm. Maybe not exactly. Maybe there's something more frightening than forgetting. *"Narrow minds devoid of imagination. Intolerance, theories cut off from reality, empty terminology, usurped ideals, inflexible systems. Those are the things that really frighten me. What I absolutely fear and loathe"* (Murakami 2005).

MARISA: Yes. I hear you. I'm not sure I'm following, though . . .

NINI: Here, let me help you. *"Through imaginal dialogue with Woolf, I was inquiring into compelling mysteries of depression with a re-vitalised spirit of curiosity and fascination; often I was surprised, when least expected, by the hidden voices in me that emerged out of the blue. My imaginary Woolf spoke in such ways 'as if' to acquaint me with the hidden, conflicted parts of the self, so we could begin to think about their meanings"* (Fang 2020).[32]

MARISA: I like that. A fictional persona connecting with you on a level that is so real it puts you in touch with a part of yourself that's so desperate to be brought to life. It reminds me of a key reason for wanting to write this book. Depression. Trauma. These topics came up in every research or knowledge-exchange public health project I embarked on over the past eight years or so, even if they weren't the topic being researched. Even if the topic was something seemingly unrelated, like non-communicable disease – smoking, drinking alcohol, unhealthy food consumption linked to obesity. Even if the topic was private-sector involvement in public health policy – tobacco, alcohol, and food industries propagating commercial determinants of health (Kickbusch, Allen, and Franz 2016). Always lurking in the background – whether interviewing corporate executives or community members in disadvantaged neighbourhoods, whether walking the streets in areas of multiple deprivation or sitting at government roundtables in developed and developing nations – were depression and trauma. It's pervasive. Individuals, communities, and systems trying to make sense of depression and trauma. Or resorting to maladaptive coping mechanisms (smoking, drinking, drugs, junk food, and so on) to try to numb or mask depression and trauma. Or companies, health services, charities, academics, policymakers, and health-care professionals trying to "fix" depression and trauma at one end of the spectrum to working with, being with, or easing the suffering that comes with depression and trauma at the other end. Depression. Trauma. It's always there in the shadows of my health research. I can't get away from it.

JUNOT DÍAZ: Yes. *"If these years have taught me anything it is this: you can never run away. Not ever. The only way out is in."*[33]

MARISA: Yes, but going "in" can be a dangerous journey, and there's no guarantee you'll end up at a place of safety. I've realised and experienced first-hand, by hearing the stories of others in my research and also being in touch with my own vulnerabilities, that trauma resists representation.

ARVA: Yes. *"Imagination, and especially the traumatic imagination, is an activity by which the human consciousness translates an unspeakable state – pain – into a readable image. The traumatic imagination uses the sublimative power of language in order to turn that which resists representation into a new and more tangible reality. Scarry considers pain and imagining 'the "framing events" within whose boundaries all other perceptual, somatic, and emotional events occur,' and then concludes that 'between the two extremes can be mapped the whole terrain of the human psyche'. I would add that between pain and imagination can be mapped the whole fictional strategy of magical realism, in which appearances are made more real than the real. However, unlike Baudrillard's depthless simulacra, oversaturated with facts and information, magical realism creates a hyperreality that is an unexplained but felt reality."*[34]

MARISA: Yes, yes, yes. It's all an illusion. The trauma. You "can't go there," so you construct this sort of escapism to deal with it . . . kind of like a journey that your mind is taking you on . . .

SONJA: *"On a journey through some new landscape of your mind . . . the landscape belongs to a racing mind and wondrous magical thoughts . . . it is a nomadic journey, where identity gains traction horizontally – fills out in a way"* (Bar-Am 2016).[35]

MARISA: Hi, Sonja. Thanks for joining us! You've arrived at a good moment for me. I was just thinking about how to explain that your particular application of magical realism is in the therapy room, with one person, working with psychosis – which, in public health terms, is at the extreme, pathologised end of *an individual making sense of reality*. How can I show that this thinking, theorising use of creative-relational, post-qualitative approaches can be applied to health research more generally? And at the population level?

[Tumbleweed.]

[Tumbleweed.]

[Tumbleweed.]

[Tumbleweed.]

[Tumbleweed.]

MARISA: Okay, something's coming to me. This is not *just* about trauma or psychosis. This is about being human. We all experience pain – it's part of the human condition – so we all need, at times, to find a way to deal with this pain when all other coping strategies we've tried are no longer helping us. Public health has very much realised that we need to include these human experiences – or what's now often referred to as the "lived experience" in research, policy, and practice – but what does that actually mean? How do you do that, practically? Methodologically? How do you incorporate a range of different, often-contradictory claims from individuals on one particular issue (say, depression) to reach a conclusion that can work at the population level? What does public health say about lived experience? And what does public health *do* with lived experience?

GRACE GATERA: *"Lived experience is what I would call 'street smarts'. The special knowledge you can only gain from going through something . . . We need active reflection and openness to confront challenges if we want to make sure that lived experience, and other conceptually similar terms, work alongside instead of replacing existing knowledge systems in mental health.*"[36]

MARISA: Yes, but it's this dialogue between these two different knowledge systems that needs unpacking. Your experience and my experience of the same (mental) health issue could be wildly different, depending on our different contexts and circumstances. Where we were born. Our traditions, rituals, religions, and cultural backgrounds. How we look, what other people see when they look at us. The languages we speak and accents we've picked up along the way. Whether we can read or write, and whether we trust the written word or see this as damning evidence of a system that's out to get us. When something is written down about us, there's a paper trail "proving" something about us. How is this data used? Who decides on how this data is interpreted and reported? How do we feel about our data being used in this way?

You know, the more I think about what it means to include "lived experience" in population health research, the more I'm left wondering how it's different to what qualitative research has always done and the argued limitations of this approach. In qualitative research, we ditch the numbers and try to figure out how people experience the world. We accept that this means we need to talk to them – gather their views, attempt to understand their beliefs, attitudes, and behaviours. We try to "evaluate human behaviour" by involving actual humans in our research rather than thinking about them as comprised of a set of variable traits that we might be able to account for. Then we report the findings, often by repeating quotes verbatim – "She said this," "They said that," "He said the other" – and that's how we breathe life into statistical datasets to include "user involvement" in clinical settings (Pathak, Jena, and Kalra 2013). We always acknowledge the limitations of this approach – personal (researcher) bias being up there with "you can't generalise or replicate this study," so what are you really adding here that's meaningful? I'm simplifying here, but quite often, we're left with the "not valid, not reliable" conundrum. A mixed-methods design analysing and integrating words and numbers might increase the rigour of a study and produce richer findings. But what does a thematic, surface-level analysis *really tell us* about the multiplicity of views and multiple realities of the people we engage with? What does this *really tell us* about what they believe to be true and how this matches up with our understanding of what is truth? How does this fit with our version of reality, and what do we do when our, or their, knowledge or reality claims don't quite fit together? And given all these incompatibilities, in what direction should public health research, practice, and policy be heading? What am I supposed to do as a public health scholar?

SARA: You game the system, that's what you do.

MARISA: Sara! What are you doing here?

SARA: Staging an intervention. You've been here before, Marisa, when you drafted your book proposal for Routledge. Think about it. Don't make me get into your head again . . .

MARISA: Well, I knew then – as I know now – that these questions are very difficult to address through linear approaches. Even the process of writing a book proposal for an academic health audience follows a particular structure, which asks for "Keywords" and a "Table of Contents" with "Chapter Abstracts." But when I'm putting forward an alternative to the "accepted reality" and knowledge generation using non-linear, post-qualitative approaches in public health – when I'm questioning the linear status quo in knowledge generation – is it possible to predict where the methodological, analytical process will go? Should I really be trying to make my book fit with this predetermined arrangement that I put forward to my publisher about a year ago? Here, let me find it . . .

Keywords: *objectivity, evidence, validity, truth, health humanities, arts-informed methods, creative methods, magical realism, ontology* (reality), *epistemology* (knowledge), *tobacco control, electronic cigarettes* (e-cigarettes), *health inequalities*

- **Table of Contents**

1. Emergence – the gap between two epistemic bubbles
2. Measuring Humanity – a methodological minefield
3. What's real and unreal in public health?
4. Knowledge is power
5. Can you hear me?
6. Convergence – accepting our differences

- **Chapter abstracts**

2.1 Emergence – the gap between two epistemic bubbles

The book begins midbreakthrough as the author, a public health policy researcher, wakes up in a vaporous, altered state of mind, body, and soul. She's literally wedged between two paradigms – public health and health humanities and arts – that have taken the form of soapy knowledge bubbles. Her first preoccupation, in her now-formless state, is to make sense of her new identity. She knows she isn't real, but what is she?

Suspended between these seemingly oppositional standpoints – and longing to be grounded – she turns to the scientific literature's understanding of realism, truth, representativeness, materiality, and corporeality alongside "other" interpretations of these concepts to see if there are overlaps in the humanities and arts. She realises that the two disciplines she's crisscrossing (and therefore her existence) have very different beliefs about "what is real and what is not." In this chapter, readers follow the author's thinking through a creative and critical literature review and analysis of

- public health's (lack of) engagement with creative methodologies and narrow conceptualisations of evidence;

- the author's ethical, ontological, and epistemological dilemmas when study-ing controversial topics in tobacco control (mostly electronic cigarettes), in particular, power and the influence of the tobacco industry to the detriment of public health;
- health humanities and arts – what it is and what it can bring to public health; and
- what magical realism is and what it can bring to public health.

By the end of Chapter 1, the author – who's now called *In-Credible* – admits she's been gaming "the system" all along. Though well-intentioned, her studies have squeezed a square peg in a round hole. Chapter 2 is her confession.

2.2 Measuring Humanity – a methodological minefield

A few years ago, In-Credible was asked by a health board to come up with a mech-anism to capture seemingly unmeasurable aspects of the human experience. This research built on her previous work with marginalised communities to improve services linked to smoking, addiction, and health more broadly. The project, now known as *Measuring Humanity*, sought to co-produce a framework with margin-alised community members and health practitioners that could systematically evaluate changes in "softer" outcomes (such as trust) linked to health, well-being, and inequalities. These aspects were to feed into more tangible, "harder" perfor-mance measures and targets saturating the health policy and practice landscape.

The approach called for innovative methods of engagement and evidence gath-ering through whatever creative or relational form was deemed valid and appro-priate for communities, be that hip-hop or theatre. Together, they endeavoured to measure health and inequalities through creativity and connectivity. And together, they stumbled into an evaluation stalemate with the very approaches we were critiquing. Working with marginalised groups, they co-produced a flex-ible, community-led framework with humanistic indicators selected and defined by community members themselves. But did this process of simplification to fulfil standard public health measurement requirements dilute or dissolve nuances that were essential to understanding the complexity of communities' experiences?

In this chapter, she reflects on the perils in attempting to measure the unmeas-urable. She troubles and interrogates key methodological concepts (see key-words) through the lens of health humanities and arts to propel public health into new territory.

2.3 What's real and unreal in public health?

Chapter 3 presents the first of three interconnected journeys that In-Credible went on while *Measuring Humanity*. Though expressed through the genre of mag-ical realism, they are all based on real-life, funded academic research projects applying the framework detailed in Chapter 2. They each engage with diverse, "disadvantaged" communities using different humanities or arts-informed meth-odologies and all collected data for health research, policy, and practice.

This story merges two framework applications: one in "aspiring communities," a project funded by the European Social Fund through the Scottish government in partnership with the charity Bethany Christian Trust; the other in "green spaces," funded by the Conservation Volunteers.

"What's real and what's unreal in public health?" centres around a Clinical Trial situated in The Community, a place where everyone has a "mental health issue." Every Community Member has been, at some point, on antidepressants or another type of medication, but their circumstances and health outcomes remain unchanged. They continue to be individually and collectively morose and over-indulging in what the experts are calling "health-damaging behaviours" – smoking, drinking, eating junk foods, and so on.

The Community is deemed a public health disaster, so experts are brought in to conduct the Straightforward Inane Lucid Liability (SILLY) Clinical Trial. They arrive in The Community (well, they don't ever step foot in The Community; they stay in their offices and labs and research it from afar) armed with a rigorous research design with all the hallmarks of a proper, credible, scientific study. But soon they discover members in The Community have gone mad. Some of them are claiming a pine marten (a furry creature from the weasel family) has been making them feel well. Others are seeking comfort and health in poetry. They contemplate bringing in a team of psychiatric nurses into The Community to assess for collective psychosis, especially when they encounter two members in The Community conducting their own study (they're not even researchers!) with the silliest of research questions: Is a poem or a pine marten better for your mental health?

This chapter unpacks and critiques ontology and competing versions of reality by following "experts" and "lay people" as they conduct the SILLY Clinical Trial and its sillier spin-off study. It introduces theories of affect to public health and links this to debates on power and positionality in research, policy, and practice. It also enacts and simultaneously illustrates how movement, the environment and environmental art, crafts, and poetry can be used as public health methodologies.

SARA: Should you really be trying to make your book fit with this predetermined arrangement that you put forward to your publisher about a year ago? No, not really. If you're going to join me in my world – in my reality – and accept knowledge in the way I'm offering it to you through my poems and my art and the art of my environment, you'll need to trust in the process of your writing. You'll need to trust in the process of my writing. You'll need to connect with the art form I present to you. You'll need to be in touch with all that is in me and all that is in you as you bear witness to my writing and my art, as you try to make sense of my writing and my art. This "act" makes you "aware that the poetic is not outside" you "but within."[37]

MARISA: So in some way, I'm an extension of the products of your creativity? An extension of your expression of your art?

SARA: Yes. It's quite a dense concept to get your head around, and the only way I know this stuff is because I've Downloaded your mind, so I know you know this stuff too. Remember that paper you read by Suely Rolnik a couple of years ago, "*Molding a Contemporary Soul: The Empty-Full of Lygia Clark*" (Rolnik 1999)? Your mind's been trying to make sense of it ever since, subconsciously. And just when you think you've grasped the key argument – just when you think you can touch the essence of that paper and Lygia's thesis[38] – you lose it. It passes.

MARISA: Yes! I feel like I know what she means when she talks about " '*the empty-full*', *the experience of the vibrating body at the moment in which the exhaustion of a cartography*[39] *is processed, when the silent incubation of a new reality of feeling is under way, that incubation being the manifestation of the fullness of life in its power of differentiation. The crises were the living of these passages, which in the artist's subjectivity took place like 'vulvanic eruptions'* " (Rolnik 1999).[40] But I also feel that as soon as I "know" this "new reality," when my "feeling" of this "new reality" "is underway," it moves somewhere else. Outside of me. Into you, maybe? Into the art? Into the world around me?

SARA: Yes. I think that's what's so magical about it. In the art world, Lygia exposed ways for people who were "viewers" of art to become "participants" of art as they interacted with her art. So her art had movement. Her art was active. Her art was activism. So her creativity was political. It was also non-threatening. It connected the individual to the system. It "*dealt with the relationship between inside and outside, and, ultimately, between self and world*" (Clark and Bois 1994). And above all, it made you feel alive. "As Clark wrote, '*Previously, man had a discovery, a language. He could use it his entire life and thus feel alive. Today, if we crystallize into a language we stop, inexorably. We totally stop expressing. It's necessary to be always catching.*' *In evoking this power in the spectator 'to be attracting' the mutations of time that manifest themselves in his or her vibrating body, Clark's work turns him or her into the missing contemporary people, to replace the modern people, those spectators of art and life, who run the risk of succumbing to the impasses of contemporary experience if they persisted in the way they organized their subjectivity. Or worse, the risk of producing irreparable damage such as the carnage we have witnessed in the name of perpetuation of supposed ethnic, religious, and national identities in a world irreversibly invaded by hybridization. In realizing the modern utopia in her work, Clark exhausted this cartography and prepared the ground for a new dream.*" (Rolnik 1999)[41]

MARISA: You know, that me reminds me of what Sonja's saying when she talks about her engagement with Eva using magical realism as a guide through the "liminal terrain" of Eva's first episode of psychosis (Bar-Am 2016).

SONJA: "As Eva was talking I started sifting through my mind, and through the reading I'd done: *Maps, maps, what direction would this dialogue take? Where would I take it? Where would Eva go with it? What is delusional may be real to Eva?*" (Bar-Am 2016)[42]

MARISA: Yes, but how to "map" that reality in a linear (enough) form to make sense to other readers, researchers, policymakers, and practitioners? Thinking about cartography is helpful. Studying, making, and utilising maps blends scientific techniques with artistic creations. It's based on the idea that reality – or what we imagine to be reality – can be represented effectively in a spatial form.

SONJA: Yes . . . *"the multiplication of realities and how to map that: psychotic and non-psychotic, not un – or super reality, but magical reality, and further how to map the contexts of these realities, a narrative that contextualises the pre- and post-psychotic identity . . ."* (Bar-Am 2016)[43]

MARISA: There is a reality "before," and a reality "after." How to map out that journey? How to move in and out of these realities using different, creative knowledge forms that are non-linear? How do you order them, in some way, to make some sort of sense out of them?

SARA: That's tricky, Marisa. Remember what one of the reviewers of your book proposal said and how you responded?

MARISA: Remind me, please?

SARA: Okay. Here's the Download . . .

Review 1

- **How much of the text will be fictional writing?**

The honest answer is, I don't know yet, and if I'm being true to the theory and methods I'm applying, I shouldn't know until the words appear on the page. This is the catch-22 when writing peer-reviewed publications on this topic for leading, conventional public health/medical journals and also funding applications that lean on traditional and linear forms of knowledge generation.

We can't predict outputs or outcomes when using these approaches. In the field, these are co-produced with participants. On paper, these emerge as the writing unfolds. I'd be gaming the methodology if I made something up.

I simply need to trust in the process and convince you, my publisher, that I will strike the appropriate balance between fictional and didactic writing. I've given the core argument a considerable amount of thought and am confident that I can make a valuable contribution to move public health in a different direction.

Elizabeth Adams St. Pierre, a leading academic on post-structural/post-modern approaches, explains how writers using this approach need to *"trust their reading to sustain them, trust the concepts they've studied that reorient their thought, and trust experimentation and creativity, which will be constituted differently in every post quali-tative study"* (St. Pierre 2018).[44]

Rajchman (2000)[45] tells us how the writing becomes the emerging and unfold-ing matter of enquiry. I need to trust my writing, trust in the process, and trust that *"something may come out, though one is not yet completely sure what."*[46]

This is a very important question, though, as I'm trying to reach and influence mainstream health scholars, many of whom will not have been exposed to this type of writing, theorising, and research design. I don't want to alienate or lose them along the way by being too progressive and post-modern, so . . .

• How will you ensure the more creative elements stay focused on the message without being too didactic? I'm thinking of a couple of books we published quite a long time ago in a totally different subject area but had a somewhat-similar approach using creative techniques to critique the field. One was excellent, but the creative parts of the other were, frankly, poorly written and overly literal. I think this balance is what the reviewer is getting at here.

I intend to take the advice I give to my MScR and PhD students, who grapple with this very issue when trying to address assessment criteria (prescriptive/ instructive) while producing creative theses that do not conform to conventional academic norms.

I suggest providing a "road map" at the start, giving the reader a heads-up of what is coming rather than plunging straight in. This preface would explain that given the non-linear approach of the creative inquiry and central argument, a conventional structure for an academic book would not work. Instead, I opt for a more fitting creative narrative, allowing different voices to speak to each other, letting them flow from one topic to the next. To give orientation to a more conservative reader, I will probably outline the key learning points at the start to show how my book would have looked in a more conventional structure.

MARISA: Yes. This seems sensible, necessary even. Introducing post-qualitative inquiry to public health is a big leap. I don't want this work to be useless to a discipline that relies on ordered thinking and methodological approaches that will "arrive at" some sort of meaningful health conclusions and recommendations. For this work to be useful, there will need to be a bridge between the "not knowing" and the "knowing." There needs to be a road map.

SARA: Yes, that would be helpful, I think. Okay, here's something to anchor you before I take you back into my reality.

MARISA: Back into your reality?

SARA: Yes. You were in Beguile with me and the rest of The Community.

MARISA: Hmm. It's been a while. What was happening again before this detour?

SARA: We'd finished our ritual, gathered on the top of a building touching the sky. And we'd just started projecting a scene on the 4DX screens of me in a room – a clinical setting maybe – with someone you appear to have recognised.

MARISA: Yes! That feels like a lifetime ago. Is that still happening?

SARA: As we speak, as you type. We'll be back there in just a moment. For now, remember the Hammock of Happiness?

MARISA: Well, I can remember In-Credible – that's what the researcher's called now, right? In-Credible. It's in my book proposal, in the Chapter Abstracts you've read. I can remember In-Credible asking you about the Hammock of Happiness as Mary lay there in an emerald-coloured sling made of fabric, a solid rope, and some netting suspended between two hardwood trees that had anchored themselves in the middle of the circle.

SARA: Correct. So you didn't make that bit up. In fact, most of that scene is informed by real experiences and real data you collected in the field on one of your projects.

MARISA: Yes, I remember it well. Here, let me find the report foreword I wrote for The Conservation Volunteers . . .

2.4 Foreword (for TCV report) – June 2018

Dr Marisa de Andrade – PI for Measuring Humanity, School of
Health in Social Science, Centre for Creative-Relational Inquiry,
University of Edinburgh

> *"I know it works because of the journey I've been on . . . but I can't prove it."*
> – TCV practitioner

A year ago, I delivered a training workshop to TCV practitioners on the Asset-Based Indicator Framework as part of *Measuring Humanity*. The participant-led research programme uses bottom-up creative community engagement to challenge policymakers and academics to reassess what counts as evidence when developing policies, practices, and recommendations.

TCV practitioners on the Wild Ways Well programme have been using the framework as an evaluation tool to explore how the green space improvement programme supports individual resilience and well-being for people who are at risk of developing a mental health condition.

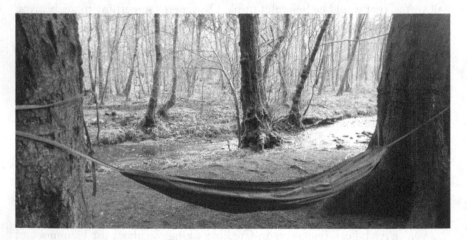

Figure 2.1 The Hammock of Happiness

Source: photograph taken during the Wild Ways Well project by the Conservation Volunteers in 2018, shared with the University of Edinburgh as data for the project *Measuring Humanity in Green Spaces*.

Findings are fascinating. Much like the other applications of *Measuring Humanity* with disadvantaged, Black Minority Ethnic, and Deaf communities, practitioners highlight the importance of using creative and relational methods to evidence wider impacts of programmes rather than rolling out the same quantitative measures. They also explain how these quantitative methods are, in some cases, inaccurately capturing the views of their participants and producing misleading results.

Environmental art, videos, reflective diaries, and photographs – of *The Hammock of Happiness*, for example – are proving to be richer, more appropriate data sources for their community members. They also open up conversations on how individuals and communities are affected by systemic issues that perpetuate ill health.

However, there is still some hesitation amongst practitioners that these count as "evidence" or "proof." This isn't surprising, given our fixation on the biomedical approach to generating and using evidence – even when this fails the most marginalised.

Creativity and the act of humans coming together in community provide missing pieces of evidence that must be understood to tackle complex health problems. *Measuring Humanity* will continue to value people's stories and lived experiences as evidence of the effectiveness of Green Health projects. It will also continue to flag up problems with traditional conceptualisations of measurement, metrics, evaluation, and evidence on this journey.

SARA: So what did you do with all that data you collected in the field for that project? Remember you reviewed the experiences of participants, the project officer, and other staff members in their approach to evaluation of the Wild Ways Well programme. . . ?

MARISA: Yes, I analysed their experiences through a framework.

SARA: Okay. And what did that tell you?

MARISA: Quite a lot about the process of evaluation and what different aspects of the human experience mean to people as they're connecting with nature and environmental art. But it threw up more questions than answers about what evaluation actually is. What evaluation actually does. What does any intervention really "prove" if you starting digging a little deeper? Do you know what I'm saying here?

SARA: Well, yes. I know all about the SILLY Clinical Trial and what "health experts" are calling its sillier spin-off study about poems and pine martens. But I think you're going to have to work a bit harder here if you want to explain what you mean to a public health audience. . .

MARISA: Okay, do you want to see a brief summary of findings from the project's participatory action research (PAR)?

SARA: Hmm . . . let me see. What word count are you on?

MARISA: For this book? 37,435.

SARA: And how many words is this book supposed to be?

MARISA: Hmm. I said in my book proposal around 70,000 words, but to be perfectly honest, I just made that up.

SARA: Okay, what does your contract with the publisher say?

MARISA: Hang on, let me check.

SARA: I think we're just wasting words now.

MARISA: No, I think this is important context. We're all about the numbers in this game . . . it helps to give us form, to give us structure . . . we need to keep our ideas and arguments focused, less rambling and loose thinking . . . but post-qualitative inquiry needs a bit more space. . .

SARA: Yeah, but you still need to keep it focused. What's the word count?

MARISA: Okay . . . here's my contract: "*(a) the complete typescript of the Work in Microsoft Word format or another recognisably generic format such as Rich Text Formatting (RTF) which will be no longer than 110,000 words (including the references, bibliography, figures, illustrations, and index).*"

SARA: Okay. It may be tight. And also, you've still got a lot of writing to do! Here's what I think. Somewhere in the book, further down the line, figure out a way to show how your framework findings in linear form *would have looked* after a surface-level analysis using thematic coding and an inductive-deductive – or an abductive – approach. This will also give you a chance to think about whether that approach really allowed you to monitor change before, during, and after the evaluations. What meaningful insights really emerged using that traditional approach to knowledge generation? So there's a plan for the future. Right now, trust in the post-qualitative process and keep pulling quotes and findings from your dataset to inform your tale of magical realism. It's time to get back now. You've abandoned me and The Community just as I was about to expose more of my vulnerabilities. And I can't even imagine how In-Credible is feeling after all this time by herself in our reality. . .

***

I, In-Credible, could hear Sara's thoughts as she spoke to this other person in her mind. That person was unmistakeably Professor Ebba. The two of them were definitely in a clinical room of some kind, their full forms replicated on the huge 4DX screens in front of me in The Futile Forest.

Reader, maybe if you come a little closer, you'll hear them too. Shhh . . .[47]

Listen. Can you hear Sara's thoughts too?

> I'm not sure if I even like Ebba. I even find her name mildly offensive, as intrusive as her manner. The Institution says her job is to stay neutral. As a health researcher – certainly an academic of this standing in scientific and clinical settings – she's completely unbiased, they say. Objectivity all the way.
>
> I beg to differ.
>
> In my mind, she's asking leading questions that will eventually open doors to answers I definitely wasn't searching for. One of these days, she'll tell me what's really gone on with me. Her findings will be published somewhere important, with a range of recommendations that are best for people like me.

People like me. People with problems. People who need to be fixed. People who had a troubled childhood.

Did you know "exposure to traumatic experiences in early life plays a significant aetiological role in a host of mental health disorders across the life course, including psychosis" (O'Neill, Maguire, and Shevlin 2021)?[48]

Aetiological – I had to look it up, do a quick online search. I don't know why they use words like that when speaking to us "lay people." Aren't they familiar with the ethics application process? Consent Forms and Participant or Patient Information Sheets should not use jargon. Explain things simply, please, for us simple people, please.

Aetiological. I like that it has two meanings. The medical one: "causing or contributing to the development of a disease or condition." And the magical one: "serving to explain something by giving a cause or reason for it, often in historical or mythical terms."[49]

There's nothing mythical about Professor Ebba – she's very real. But there's something about her eyes that remind me of ice-blue marbles somehow floating in a glass of milk. I hate milk, unless it comes from a coconut.

Something about her translucent skin that evokes flashbacks from childhood of white rabbits (not the cotton-tail kind that are now extinct, but the insipid sweets with pictures of white rabbits and edible wrappers).

And I hated my childhood.[50] Well, I think I hated my childhood. These days, it's difficult to remember what I may have forgotten, difficult to forget what I don't want to remember, though some shapeless memories remain. Like this one, from my childhood, shoving its way in to the here and now as I'm trying to focus on Professor Ebba. This one, of the ginger cat (whose name I've forgotten, but I'm going to go with Muggles) appearing on our doorstep four years on the trot on Christmas Eve, back when people shared holidays and homes and hearts. Back in the days of The Family Unit.

Back in the room.

Yes, I'm not sure if I like Professor Ebba. There's something about her "expert" voice that jars with her "Hello, I'm here to listen to you and take your views seriously" voice.

But she's here to listen to me. The Institution's handpicked me for the Patient and Public Involvement Group (we like to call it PIG) on the SILLY Trial, so I'm one of the lucky "service users" who get to have their say in the field of mental health research (that's how they're saying it).

At first, I felt like I was a part of the main picnic – you know that popular group that was too cool for high school, the one everyone love-hates, the one everyone wants to be a part of. I felt important. I felt like I was being heard when I spoke about the troubles of my past, the struggles of my present, my fear of the future.

Then something changed inside of me. Something didn't feel quite right. Still, I kept on going. Reluctantly opening up more and more each session.

The protocol for the study says we each need to meet the Principal Investigator, Professor Ebba, by ourselves once every two weeks in a clinic none of us had ever heard of before this all started. It's about an hour away from Beguile, in a twenty-seven-floor glass building shaped like a cucumber.

I've never seen anything like this place before in my life. Fancy. *This is how the other half live*, I think to myself every time I arrive and get swiped through high-level security with finger and iris scans.

Etched 'round the rounded erection in a bold black are the letters V-E-R-I-T-A-S.[51] The company that's funded the research. The company that funds all research. The company that owns our Uploads and Downloads. The company that owns our Highs and Lows.

The Institution pays for our e-taxis there and back and also throws in lunch and some expenses – so it's a no-brainer, really. Plus, we get to pour out our hearts and souls to the immaculate Professor, who makes all the right noises. She has a knack for smoothing your surfaces. Stripping off your edges.

I find myself complaining about everything and everyone who had ever wronged me, and it feels good. She keeps telling me that's the point of these sessions. Let it all out until there's nothing left but a vacuous hole of nothingness. Emptiness. Pointlessness.

It took me a while to trust her, to open up. On day 1, I could feel my fists clenching when she said stupid things like, "That sounds quite frightening" or "Tell me about the dreams you had last night and the memories that keep upsetting you."

Utterly clichéd, but I swear she's still using these turns of phrase even though we no longer need to hold on to our patchy thoughts and sketchy memories. Even though they're all literally being stored for us in the Sphere-Blue Drive to "free up headspace for augmented thinking and superior sensing," as the marketing slogan says.

I stare past Professor Ebba's sleek hair. "When was the last time my head popped into hyper-reality mode? When I saw life as it truly is?"

She nods.

This doesn't need much thought. "This morning. When I got in the shower." My skin recoils as it recalls the scalding from the rainstorm replicated in my avocado bathroom that hasn't been upgraded since the seventies (the showerhead is broken, as is the toilet seat).

I don't want to tell her anything, but it all comes pouring out. Words lashing out of the outlets in my mind, looking for a new place to live.

"I was running late, so I reached for my toothpaste so I could brush my teeth in the shower while conditioner washed out of my hair. And that was when I saw the words that had been right in front of my face ever since the day I bought this brand of toothpaste because it was buy-one-get-one-free at Mega-Med. I guess I've been using it for about . . . well, at least . . . well, 'round about the time of my last Upload and Firmware Upgrade, so thirteen days, I guess. Thirteen days I've been blindly staring at a tube that says, 'Cleansing crystals to control those cavities before they've even seen light of day!' and only today, on day 14, does the penny drop. Only today do I see the link between my toothpaste and what's going on around us. It's like someone's turned a switch on or given me a pair of glasses that focuses my vision and crystallises my thinking. And then I'm flying. Free associating. Like mind acrobatics. Leaping from thought to thought, connecting the dots, making sense of it all."

"Sense of what all? I guess I'm struggling to follow what you're saying, Sara."

I resist the urge to punch her in the face. She's part of the problem. I'm screaming inside; I can hear my head giving me instructions to shout until I'm blue in the face.

I take a deep breath.

"I'm saying, Professor Ebba, that it's all connected. None of this is just happening. It's all carefully planned to perfection. Everything going on in my head, in your head, in everyone's head, is controlled. But it's so subtle, so beautifully created that it's almost impossible to wrap your head around. Well, you can't wrap your head around it because apparently there's no room left in your head full stop. Or at least not enough space to think big or feel good, or at least that's what they've told you. So they tell you that and then you believe them and actually pay them your hard-earned cash – so they're winning twice! – to hold your thoughts and memories and all that other grey stuff in some vapour-type virtual container that doesn't even exist in the real world. And while the tragedy appears to be that they're free to do whatever they choose with this matter, the real tragedy is that we've simply handed our matter over to them as if they were Buddhist monks on an impoverished alms round. Like Buddhist monks with empty bowls, begging for the basics, just to stay alive. We've given away our total freedom. This, Professor Ebba, is the tragedy."

I can hear her fingers tapping a screen as I speak. Selectively inputting sound bites from my stream of consciousness as if she's some superhuman id-superego diffusor. *Tip tap.* According to the time being projected on the wall, I've been lying here for two hours, fourteen minutes, and fifty-nine seconds already. Long enough to have figured out her patterns. She says nothing for an abnormally long time while I stare at the fluorescent lampshade hanging from the bright white ceiling. *Tip tap.* And just when I'm just about ready to break the silence with a tangential tale, to comment on the brightness of the light of the white of the ceiling, of the tapping of the fingers, just when I'm just about ready to attack the silence with a scream to distract me from the darkness of the brightness, she gently nudges me.

"All this from your toothpaste. That must be frightening."

"Frightening, no. Infuriating, yes." *Tip tap.*

"Infuriating? Huh." Another nudge. And then the silence. Into the brightness. Into my darkness. I'm tired. So utterly exhausted.

"Sara." Silence.

"Sara?"

"What?"

"How are you feeling?"

"Feeling?" I start biting my nails.

I wonder if this is some kind of trick. What am I supposed to say?

We don't feel anymore – well, that's what they tell us. Ever since The Tipping Point, they've regulated our feelings through Emotion-Defibrillators ©, tiny implants that each law-abiding citizen has right near their heart.

Unprecedented technology, they told us. What we all need to cope with reality these days.

It'll help us, they told us. To feel pleasure again. To offset the unbearable pain that arrived on the day that it all became too much and we tipped into mass dissociation.

It's a normal defence mechanism, they told us, to switch off from reality when a person can't cope during a traumatic time. The trouble was, they told us, we were all still acting and living as if we were in the trauma when the truth was, they told us, it was over.

Our environment was no longer traumatic, they told us; everything was back to normal. But we weren't getting on with it, they told us, as they trialled a device first in mice then in humans in controlled environments, then in humans in uncontrolled environments.

"Eureka, it works!" they told us.

Then it became the law.

Suddenly, humans feeling again. Their emotions tweaked, kept in balance by the Emotion-Defibrillator © through some kind of mind-body interface with the Sphere-Blue Drive.

I'm biting my nail so hard now that my cuticle is bleeding. I've been quiet for too long that I have to say something before she gets suspicious.

"I'm feeling exactly as I should. Totally balanced."

"Hmm." Silence.

"Sara, you've been having these thoughts for so long I can only imagine how exhausting it must be. I see here from your records that you're on antidepressants for anxiety, depression, and psychosis. How do you feel about upping your dose?" I wait for the *tip tap*. Silence.

I raise her silence with silence.

"Sara, how do you feel about upping your dose?"

A rage starts bubbling inside me. I can feel it fermenting as I think of all the things I could say and how I could say them. Someone's screaming in my head. *ARE YOU SERIOUS? HAVEN'T YOU BEEN LISTENING TO A WORD I'VE BEEN SAYING?* I spot a moth blind itself in the bulb.

"I could think of nothing worse," I say through gritted teeth. "I'm on to something here. Things have been speeding up since they were slowed down by Veritas Inc. You know that. I know that. We're going faster and faster, and I'm trying to make sense of it all. Not just for me, not just for The Community. For everyone. There's a lot of work to be done, and I don't want to be numbed out."

Tip. Tap.

"Sara, I believe it's time for you to up your dose."

"Have you been listening to a single word I've been saying? The Community needs me more than ever before. The world needs me more than ever before. This is no time for more drugs."

"I hear you, Sara, I really do. You aren't the expert here, though."

ARE YOU KIDDING ME! I THOUGHT I WAS A PIG PERSON BECAUSE I AM THE EXPERT!

"Trust me."

"Thanks, but no thanks." I start getting up, ready to march out the door.

"Sara, it's a Protective Order."

I freeze. I've never been given one of those before. I know better than to push back, to ask questions, to do anything other than lie there quietly. Passively.

"Will that fix me?" I want to ask sarcastically. "Please tell me that'll fix me," I want to say sincerely. I feel myself becoming belligerent but don't want to be. I'm just tired. So, so tired.

Her chair creaks. I hear her stand up. Time must be up.

"We'll pick up next time, Sara. Until then, take care. Pick up your prescription on the way out, please."

She walks out before we can connect. I'm left to unclench my fists and straighten my black polyester-cotton dress. I put on my boots, straighten my back, and drag myself out the door.

It's 5:00 p.m. I feel lost.

The street's steaming when I step on to it. The skies seemingly split during my PIG session to spit out a week's worth of rain that had been accumulating in the bellies of dark, pregnant clouds. As I scamper across the intersection, dodging terrestrial e-Charges that are driving themselves to programmed destinations, I'm suddenly smacked by the mental image of me with a bump, swollen and miserable. Me with a bump, swollen and happy as I rub my unborn child with my nurturing palm.

A wave of nausea washes over me. Phantom nausea to match the phantom pregnancy in my mind. I run after an e-Taxi that's dropping off three strangers. Everything feels strange.

It's been almost ten years. Almost a decade since they did away with it. Did away with the concept of conception under the Abundant Infertility Act. I can't stop thinking about it. How can the banishment of birth be hailed as the most progressive policy of its time?[52]

Time.

Time moves forward; it never moves back. [Rule # 1]

Thirty seconds later, another e-Taxi fails to notice the puddle where the street meets the sidewalk and soaks me as I get into my transporter.

I speed away, but I'm not going fast enough. I race through the options in my mind. Too many dead ends. I need to get away from here. Fast. I need.

To. Get.

Away from here. Fast.

I do what I do best in moments like these. I think of words that may or may not be related and put them together in sequence that may or may not be repetitive.

I let my mind hop from word to word, trusting in the words that will arrive in some form that will help me understand what's going on inside. Some call this poetry.

TRUTH-REALITY-KNOWLEDGE-MADNESS[53]

They told me I was a crazy, and I believed them, because I thought I once was.
Then I climbed my way through, climbed my way up. And even then
– at the top of my mountain –
they reminded me of that time.
Those people. The ones who diagnose, treat, manage.
Those people. The ones who help.
Those people. The ones you love.
Is it okay to break down and get some help
if your records will always show you once couldn't
Help
Yourself?
The only way out is through.
And so I start on the way in.
At the beginning of life, perhaps.
Or the lives before mine.
Then later.
In pain. Trauma. Worming my way through loss.
A baby stuck outside a womb's wall.
My walls are impenetrable.
They threw me inside a torture chamber.
Exposed at the intersection of mind meeting The Powers that be.
I was never crazy.
I might as well have been.
They threw their people under a bus. The ones with red tape who
Blamed
Me.
The ones we loved more than life itself.
Under the bus, we were dragged. Kicking and screaming along the path of most resistance,
until we came to a grounding halt.
Prove it.
Prove you aren't mad.
Prove you are sane.
Prove it?

I have nothing to prove.

Help me make sense of reality when the world's gone mad.

When you know you are well but "proof" points and shoves and kicks and throws you

against a wall of

Shame.

Imagine you don't have anything to prove.

Nothing at all.

Imagine you're still asked to prove it.

Imagine this whole shock show is a

Sham.

– Sara

I'm flying away.

I need to fly away.

In a few hours, I will be flying away.

Notes

1 Page 20.
2 Page 24.
3 Page 37.
4 This thinking is once again influenced by Spindler.
5 Distinct from medical humanities with its biomedical gaze, the emergent discipline of health humanities is "more inclusive, outward-facing and applied" and engages with "contributions of those marginalized" (Crawford et al. 2010) (page 1). It seeks to challenge the dominance of medicalisation by pushing against or opening up boundaries in health care by valuing the humanities and arts to produce new meanings of health and illness through (co-produced) creative engagements. It connects with multiple disciplines such as anthropology, law, literature, drama, and music to conceptualise and apply humanities and arts in health care as healing, methodology, and explorations on the human condition (Crawford et al. 2010, 2015).
6 (Crawford et al. 2015) citing (Ross, Schroeder, and Ness 2013) (page 26).
7 Page 1.
8 Page 5.
9 Page 227.
10 Page 228.
11 This story – and variations of it – has been told to me by various Community Members about their personal experiences or the experiences of other Community Members around them.
12 Wow, eleven months already. Time. It really does move forward; it never moves back.
13 Page 381.
14 Ibid.
15 Ibid.
16 Page 85.
17 Page 387.
18 Ibid.
19 Page 137.

20 Page 75.
21 I'm once again thinking about *insight* as both a clinical term in mental health and also the innate ability one has to accurately know things. To truly understand the core or essence of something. To live with awareness of internal and/or external realities (see Chapter 1).
22 Karen Barad's concept of "spacetimemattering" refers to an entangled "ongoing flow of agency" with all its constituent parts as entwined and communally constituting, even space and time as indivisible "spacetime" (Barad 2007) (pages 140–223). In *Arts of Living on a Damaged Planet*, Karen describes the concept as "a set of static points, coordinates of a void, but a dynamism of différancing" (Barad 2017) (page G110).
23 Here I'm reflecting on the Freudian structural theory: the preconscious state that "sits" between the unconscious and conscious state where we are sensing something or parts of ourselves but we are not (yet) fully aware of it (Freud 1961). A bit like [Rule # 2]: follow the sun. I'm not sure where the sun is taking me, but I'm compelled to follow it as if it's some inner compass.
24 The experiences of community members – as they've retold them and I've experienced and reimagined them here – are influenced by "posthuman thinking and theorising" that "teaches us that we have to think about bodies, all bodies, human and nonhuman in relationality. It is not enough to talk only and in isolation about human bodies." Gale and Wyatt (2018) question, "What can a body do? What work does a particular performance or act do? We are impelled to bring nonhuman as well as human bodies into these relationalities . . . must come to terms with the rhetoric of Spinoza that says that all bodies, human and nonhuman, have the capacity to affect and be affected" (pages 566–7).
25 Inspired by the Native American song "Fly Like an Eagle." Origins of the song not found despite heavy online searching.
26 These words are inspired by a pagan chant, "Round and Round We Dance." Similar to "Fly Like an Eagle," it was difficult to track information on the official origins of the chant.
27 Page 60.
28 There have also been various interpretations of Murakami's work drawing on influential academics such as Jacque Derrida and Julia Kristeva.
29 Page 1.
30 As it happens, I could easily have had a conversation like this with Nini as we're colleagues in the same subject area and Associate Directors at the Centre for Creative-Relational Inquiry at the University of Edinburgh. But what's so imaginative about that?
31 Page 14.
32 Ibid.
33 This is author Junot Díaz speaking. He quotes from his magical realism novel *The Brief Wondrous Life of Oscar Wao* (Díaz 2007).
34 I'm citing here the works of Eugene L. Arva's, an English Literature scholar with an MFA in Creative Writing and Fiction whose research focuses on magical realism in literature and film, contemporary theory, Holocaust studies, trauma theory, postcolonial studies, American cinema, and film philosophy (Arva 2008) (pages 164–65).
35 Page 7.
36 Grace is a Lived Experience consultant in mental health at the Wellcome Trust (Gatera 2021).
37 Drawn from the writing of Lygia Clark published in the 2014 book *Lygia Clark: The Abandonment of Art 1948–1988* (Butler and Pérez-Oramas 2014).
38 The Brazilian artist Lygia Clark was connected to the Brazilian Constructivist movements of the mid-twentieth century. Along with other artists and poets, she cofounded the Neo-Concrete movement exploring novel artistic conceptualisations of utopian capital inspired by cybernetics, gestalt psychology, and the optical illusions. The artists wanted "greater sensuality, colour and poetic feeling in concrete art" (Almino 2015).

39 Studying, making, and utilising maps – cartography – blends scientific techniques with artistic creations, maps. As a discipline, it's based on the idea that reality – or what we imagine to be reality – can be represented effectively in a spatial form.

40 Page 5.

41 Page 25.

42 Page 6.

43 Ibid.

44 Page 12.

45 Page 7.

46 That's a lot of trust. How would one measure that on a scale?

47 Trust in this magical realist device of turning to *"illusion and magic as a matter of survival in a civilization priding itself on scientific accomplishments, positivist thinking, and the metaphysical banishment of death."* Trust that *"the falsehood"* of this *"fantastic imagery [is] exactly in order to expose the falsehood – and the traumatic absence – of the reality that it endeavors to re-present"* (Arva 2008) (page 61).

48 Page 2.

49 Definitions given from *Bing* online search engine.

50 According to O'Neill, Maguire, and Shevlin (2021), people who've experienced recent trauma self-regulate through dissociation, and this increases the risk of experiencing symptomatic psychosis. Childhood and adulthood traumas feed into "many dissociative accounts of the trauma – hallucination relationship" (page 433).

51 The truth, in Latin.

52 Some of the Community Members I connected with spoke of traumas associated with the one-child policy in China from 1979 to 2015 to curb an explosive population growth. The policy was enforced by the government through a range of incentives and sanctions such as forced abortions and sterilisations.

53 Poetry was used as a means of data collection in some of the aspiring communities. A community worker noted, "It's hard to articulate a story like [Sara's] without using poetry or something to capture the real depth of what that conversation was like. . . . At the end of that conversation what you end up writing down in your notes is something like, 'Met [Sara], she answered this, this is the question she picked, and she has skills in. . .,' but the real power of that conversation is something I think you hold as a worker yourself. . . . It's hard to put that into a report. . . . You can't really capture the power of that moment because it's so human. It's just so fleeting. It's just what happened with that group of four people" (de Andrade 2018).

References

Aldea, Eva. 2011. *Magical Realism and Deleuze: The Indiscernibility of Difference in Postcolonial Literature. Magical Realism and Deleuze: The Indiscernibility of Difference in Postcolonial Literature.* Bloomsbury Academic. https://doi.org/10.5040/9781472542601.

Almino, Elisa Wouk. 2015. "Contemporary Brazilian Artists at Home with Neo-Concrete Movement." *Art Miami Magazine.* 2015. https://artmiamimagazine.com/neo-concrete/.

Arva, Eugene L. 2008. "Writing the Vanishing Real: Hyperreality and Magical Realism." *Journal of Narrative Theory* 38: 74–78. www.jstor.org/stable/41304877.

Bar-Am, Sonja. 2016. "First Episode Psychosis: A Magical Realist Guide Through Liminal Terrain." *Australian and New Zealand Journal of Family Therapy* 37 (3): 381–96. https://doi.org/10.1002/ANZF.1159.

Barad, Karen. 2007. "Meeting the Universe Halfway: Quantum Physics and the Entanglement of Matter and Meaning." *Meeting the Universe Halfway:* 140–223. https://doi.org/10.1215/9780822388128.

———. 2017. "No Small Matter: Mushroom Clouds, Ecologies of Nothingness, and Strange Topologies of SpaceTimeMattering." *Arts of Living on a Damaged Planet*

(January): G103–20. www.academia.edu/39975279/No_Small_Matter_Mushroom_
Clouds_Ecologies_of_Nothingness_and_Strange_Topologies_of_SpaceTimeMattering.

Butler, Cornelia, and Luis Pérez-Oramas. 2014. *Lygia Clark: The Abandonment of Art, 1948–1988*. New York: Museum of Modern Art.

Clark, Lygia, and Yve-Alain Bois. 1994. "Nostalgia of the Body." *October* 69. https://doi.org/10.2307/778990.

Crawford, Paul, Brian Brown, Charley Baker, Victoria Tischler, and Brian Abrams. 2015. "Health Humanities." *Health Humanities*: 1–19. https://doi.org/10.1057/9781137282613_1.

Crawford, Paul, Brian Brown, Victoria Tischler, and Charley Baker. 2010. "Health Humanities: The Future of Medical Humanities?" *Mental Health Review Journal* 15 (3). https://doi.org/10.5042/MHRJ.2010.0654/FULL/XML.

de Andrade, Marisa de. 2018. "Measuring Humanity in Marginalised Communities – The Health Foundation." *The Health Foundation*. 2018. www.health.org.uk/blogs/measuring-humanity-in-marginalised-communities#:~:text=The project%2C now known as Measuring Humanity%2C sought,as trust%29 linked to health%2C wellbeing and inequalities.

Deleuze, Gilles, and Félix Guattari. 2000. *Anti-Oedipus. Capitalism and Schizophrenia*. Minneapolis: University of Minnesota Press.

Díaz, Junot. 2007. *The Brief Wondrous Life of Oscar Wao*. New York: Riverhead Books.

Fang, Nini. 2020. "Imaginal Dialogue as a Method of Narrative Inquiry." *Narrative Inquiry* 30 (1): 41–58. https://doi.org/10.1075/NI.18045.FAN/CITE/REFWORKS.

Faris, Wendy B. 2004. *Ordinary Enchantments: Magical Realism and the Remystification of Narrative*. Vanderbilt University Press. https://books.google.com/books/about/Ordinary_Enchantments.html?id=M2StyqHK2I4C.

Freud, Sigmund. 1961. *The Ego and the Id: The Standard Edition of the Complete Psychological Works of Sigmund Freud*. Edited by J. Strachey. Vol. 19. London: Hogarth Press.

Gale, Ken, and Jonathan Wyatt. 2018, "Autoethnography and Activism: Movement, Intensity and Potential." *Qualitative Inquiry* 25 (6): 566–568. https://doi.org/10.1177/1077800418800754

Gatera, Grace. 2021. "Let's Talk about Lived Experiences of Mental Health Challenges." *Wellcome Trust*. 2021. https://wellcome.org/news/lets-talk-about-lived-experiences-mental-health-challenges.

Kickbusch, Ilona, Luke Allen, and Christian Franz. 2016. "The Commercial Determinants of Health." *The Lancet Global Health* 4 (12): e895–96. https://doi.org/10.1016/S2214-109X(16)30217-0.

Mearns, Dave, and Mick Cooper. 2005. *Working at Relational Depth in Counselling and Psychotherapy*. London: Sage Publications.

Merriam-Webster. 2022. "amok." www.merriam-webster.com/dictionary/amok.

Murakami, Haruki. 2005. *Kafka on the Shore*. Edited by A. Alfred Knopf. New York: Random House.

O'Neill, Tara, Aaron Maguire, and Mark Shevlin. 2021. "Sexual Trauma in Childhood and Adulthood as Predictors of Psychotic-like Experiences: The Mediating Role of Dissociation." *Child Abuse Review* 30 (5): 431–43. https://doi.org/10.1002/CAR.2705.

Pathak, Vibha, Bijayini Jena, and Sanjay Kalra. 2013. "Qualitative Research." *Perspectives in Clinical Research* 4 (3): 192. https://doi.org/10.4103/2229-3485.115389.

Pierre, Elizabeth A. St. 2018. "Post Qualitative Inquiry in an Ontology of Immanence." 25 (1): 3–16. https://doi.org/10.1177/1077800418772634.

Rajchman, John. 2000. "The Deleuze connections." https://philpapers.org/rec/RAJTDC.

Rolnik, Suely. 1999. "Molding a Contemporary Soul: The Empty Full of Lygia Clark." In *The Experimental Exercise of Freedom: Lygia Clark, Gego, Mathias Goeritz, Helio Oiticica and Mira Schendel.* Los Angeles, CA: Museum of Contemporary Art.

Ross, Colin A., Elizabeth Schroeder, and Laura Ness. 2013. "Dissociation and Symptoms of Culture-Bound Syndromes in North America: A Preliminary Study." 14 (2): 224–35. https://doi.org/10.1080/15299732.2013.724338.

Sanders, Pete, Alan. Frankland, and Paul. Wilkins. 2009. *Next Steps in Counselling Practice: A Students' Companion for Degrees, HE Diplomas and Vocational Courses.* Herefordshire: PCCS Books.

Spindler, William. 1993. "Magic Realism: A Typology." *Forum for Modern Language Studies* XXIX (1): 75–85. https://doi.org/10.1093/FMLS/XXIX.1.75.

Williams, Matt. 2010. "What Is Planck Time?" *Universe Today.* 2010. www.universetoday.com/79418/planck-time/.

3 Measuring Humanity – a methodological mine(mind)field

***

INTERLUDE – POETRY, SCIENCE, AND SCIENCE FICTION

It's 3:00 a.m. and I can't sleep. Something is stirring inside me as I write this truthful tale of magical realism. Something is bothering me. I sense there's an answer out there – or in here – but right now, I can't figure out what it is or where it is. Instead, I start listening to a podcast, *Poetry Unbound*. I've become very fond of it; it's beautiful, "an immersive exploration of a single poem, guided by poet and theologian, Pádraig Ó Tuama. Short and unhurried; contemplative and energizing."[1]

I'm instantly drawn into a captivating episode exploring Elizabeth Bishop's poem called "Sestina," which, thanks to *Poetry Unbound*, I now know to be a typically unrhymed, intricate French verse arrangement comprised of six stanzas of six lines each and a three-line triplet. The last words of the first verse are repeated in an altered order as end words in each of the succeeding five verses. The final stanza holds all six words, two in each line, cited in the middle and at the end of the three lines.

That's a lot of technical information, and that last paragraph will probably need a few re-reads and a practical application before being fully taken in, but I share it here as it reminds me of the level of detail needed for replicating studies in the health journals I've published in.

Methodology, analysis, analytical procedure, generalisability, reproducibility. Having the same form and structure, with clear instructions on how to repeat it, certainly helps to get peer-reviewed papers published in public health.

But this isn't a scientific paper; this is a poem with the same name as a form of poetry, which was in fact renamed by the poet. The podcast narrator tells me that it was originally called "Early Sorrow," and while Pádraig admits that he doesn't know why Elizabeth changed the name, he takes an educated guess: "Bishop was a private person, so maybe she thought that 'Early Sorrow' was a little bit too obvious a title, and perhaps a little bit too close to the bone a title" (Poetry Unbound 2020).

DOI: 10.4324/9781003196488-3

His words pique me.

The hours pass. I toss and I turn, and I can't shake the image of a sorrow that's come too soon. And what does the narrator mean "a little too close to the bone"? I listen to Pádraig's lyrical voice over and over again, trying to decipher how the poem prophesises about sowing seeds to a future filled with sadness (Bishop 1956).

Now I'm wide awake, and I'm looking up the transcription of the podcast. Intrigued. It's nowhere near daybreak, winter in Scotland, though I'm anticipating my pre-schooler will wake me soon. Outside is a blanket of black with a dot of white. Life feels still. Brimming. Everything seems so full of possibilities.

For a moment, I'm in touch with this poet's loss – with the universal feeling of loss – so profoundly. Guided by Pádraig, I'm with Elizabeth when she was a child or Elizabeth's character in the poem, who is a child, drawing a house that looks like a prison in my head.

I can feel her sadness. I can feel my sadness.

A shiver.

What does this child know that I don't?

Pádraig explains her childhood trauma, her mother's institutionalisation. Her love for poetry. Her rise to Poet Laureate. Pulitzer Prize. National Book Award.

As my mind draws pictures with the six keywords in her poem, I meet that little child in her house with her grandmother by the stove. I do a web search for "almanac" – "a book published every year that includes information for that year such as important days, times of the sun rising and going down, or changes in the moon."[2]

I check the calendar. It's a full moon. A lunar eclipse, and once again I'm moved by the tides and drawn to my laptop in the middle of the night.

I am moved to tears.

I invite you now to listen to this episode of *Poetry Unbound* and see what it does to you.

Go ahead. I'll be here when you get back, then a few hours after that, I'll be teaching a two-hour-long postgraduate seminar on Humanities and Arts-Informed Methods in the Social Sciences. For the past nine weeks, almost fifty masters and PhD students from Social Research, Global Mental Health, Law, Nursing, Sports Sciences, Counselling, Curating Practices, Health in Social Sciences, and other disciplines have arrived in the real lecture room or simulated Zoom Room simultaneously to take part in what has been one of the highlights of my academic career to date.

I synchronously teach virtually so PhD Distance students or those on their fieldwork can join through a virtual classroom. Interactions between "real" and "virtual" classrooms – which include "live" group work across multiple platforms and time zones – are inspiring.

In a few hours, we will be exploring the use of poetry in research, drawing extensively on Rosie Stenhouse's work as a mental health nurse using poems to "present the 'essence' of an experience, showing rather than telling, igniting the imagination of the reader who recognises his/her own experience in the lines" (Stenhouse 2013).[3]

Rosie's contribution to the course reminds us of poetry's power to question power. To question the power imbalances in the researcher-researched voice. To harness that power to "decentre" the researcher's voice (Stenhouse 2014; Richardson 1990). To be acutely aware of the researcher's emotional entanglement with participants' experiences, and the ethical implications of speaking with rather than on behalf of participants (Owton 2017).

I have a feeling that engaging with Rosie's poetry and materials in class is going to be a powerful experience. I'm still buzzing from an incredible, collaborative session three weeks ago which, with my students' permission, will appear somewhere in this book as an experiential exploration of ethics, ontology, and epistemology in action.

The moon peeks out from behind dark clouds. As I stare at this stunning cosmological specimen, I realise that I've been here before. I have a distinct feeling of déjà vu.

This moment, I've already written it. I've already submitted it to my publisher, Routledge, in November 2020. It's been accepted for publication, and my manuscript is due in three months.

This moment, it's happening now, and I've already imagined it and written it, in the form of sample writing submitted with my book proposal, nine months ago:

"VALIDATING THE FEELS": PUBLIC HEALTH MEETS MAGICAL REALISM, HEALTH HUMANITIES, AND ARTS [WORKING TITLE – TBC]

Marisa de Andrade

<u>*A Note on Notes:*</u>[4]

"*Both science and art have to do with ordered*[5] *complexity.*"

– Lancelot Law Whyte

"*The intuitive mind is a sacred gift and the rational mind is a faithful servant. We have created a society that honours the servant and has forgotten the gift.*"[6]

– Albert Einstein

3.1 Emergence – the gap between two epistemic bubbles

It happened in the middle of the night just as the Flower Supermoon bloomed.[7] It was May, sometime in The Future. I felt shifty between the bedsheets. Troubled. Something spectacular was on the cusp of Becoming.[8] I could feel it. It was a birth. It was a death.

An enlightenment unceremoniously ushered in by a fluorescent glow that flowed in me, through me, onto the memory foam beneath me. I looked for my edges but couldn't find them. I knocked my knuckles together but couldn't hear them.

At once, I knew what had transpired on this lunular moment in time. I'd become transparent. I'd say invisible, but my body neither absorbed nor scattered nor reflected the moon rays. I was definitely perceivable – perceptible if you paid enough attention.[9] But I felt invisible.[10]

I was lodged between two epistemic bubbles.

A pair of echo chambers[11] separated my once-solid, now-spongy sides. If this were a Venn diagram, I'd be the overlap. But there's no meeting in the middle. No connection between the two. Just me, suspended between these conflicting paradigms.

I try to make sense of my new existence in this liminal space.[12] Neither here nor there, though both here and there. The one side credible. The other incredible. The one side real. The other unreal. The one side valid. The other invalid.

Objective. Subjective.

Truth. Fiction.

Science. Humanities.

Science fiction. Being human.

My boundaries become blurred.

Confusion makes way for clarity.

My mind can think *with* both sides so clearly, while my new, free-flowing form fills each chamber from the inside out. Sensing them, knowing them, becoming them.

On the one side, public health ensconced in the stability and safety of science. The other, a troubled, imposter health humanities and arts (not even an established discipline)[13] trying to be heard in a world favouring statistics.

Am I the referee? Is my role to pull them apart, kicking and screaming, as they hurl intellectual insults at each other: *"You call yourself a Public Health academic with a sample of two?"*

Or is this a story of coming together? Of meeting in the middle so public health can get in touch with the creative, intangible aspects of the human experience to produce more meaningful data? To understand what it's really like to live on the margins?

To be powerless.

Silent.

Invisible.

I feel it's the latter, and I know these creative approaches shouldn't be exclusively reserved for or *used on* the powerless, the silent, and the invisible. They could, and should, be *applied with* those within and outside the academy, at all levels of the Power Pyramid – from policymakers to professors to those who live in poverty.

We can enrich each other if we settle these two paradigms side by side. Like darkness and light, neither exists alone.

But five minutes into my mission and I'm losing my nerve. I'm reading and re-reading the words that will appear (are appearing) in this book (time swirls in this liminal space), and already I'm doubting whether it's possible to convince the sceptics.

I float out of bed, ghostlike, just as the day breaks with a crack in my consciousness. I need to get it down before this disappears into an abyss of administration. An inbox brimming with bureaucracy lies before me, but I won't get distracted.

With a hole in my stomach and a muse in my mind, I sit down at my makeshift desk (a TV tray) and begin to map out my methodological, epistemological, ontological, and ethical research journey to date. I take a sip of the strong black coffee that steams beside me (this is my reality; I get all the coffee I want).

My path has been-is[14] anything but linear. Mostly fragmented. Different parts of myself placed into and projected onto different places, different populations, different projects, different disciplines.

The academy is obsessed with interdisciplinary research with "impact," so making the case that public health and health humanities and arts can work together like a knife and fork shouldn't be impossible. But as I cut my buttered toast into triangles, I admit to myself that it feels like a distant dream.

Where to start?

3.2 Uncomfortable competing truths

I think back on my research in tobacco control and how I found myself trapped in this conflicting space for the first time in 2015 when leading a study on the role of corporate power in electronic cigarettes (e-cigarettes). I feel sick thinking about it now. Wash away the distaste in my mouth with some caffeine.

On the surface of it, I was doing what I had always done since becoming a researcher – interviewing stakeholders; analysing business, media, and policy documents; thematically coding, triangulating, presenting findings; concluding.

This time round, I felt silenced. Scared even. This was the first time I was *allowed to* speak to tobacco executives. In fact, I was told that I *should* speak to these corporate giants.[15]

The decision split public health experts. Some thought this was appalling – feeding into public relations rhetoric and lip service. Others thought this was entirely necessary. Times were a-changing, aha! Perhaps there was a product that could completely revolutionise tobacco control and stop smokers from smoking (though the fact that tobacco multinationals were heavily invested in the e-cigarette market was unfortunate).

Doing business alongside cigarette companies were the "independents" – companies without any ties to the tobacco industry – with different motivations and business strategies (de Andrade et al. 2020).

Our study was positioned smack-bang in the middle of this scientific feud that played out very publicly on the (digital) pages of leading medical journals, front pages of tabloids, and social media platforms. The retweet became synonymous with slander. If you had an opinion on e-cigs and dared to declare it through the Twitter megaphone, best you don some body armour and prepare for attack from every angle. Everyone had an opinion. And each opinion came with a unique, often-contradictory, evidence-based argument.

Many public health scholars, especially early-career researchers who were caught in the middle of this highly emotive extravaganza, quietly exited tobacco control through the backstage door (Lucherini 2018). Life's too short to be tap-dancing on the defensive all the time. Besides, publishing on e-cigarettes was increasingly challenging due to the politics of it all – and we all need those four-star Research Excellence Framework (REF) papers to be decent, credible academics these days.[16]

I pause for a moment and stare at my screen. Take a deep breath, recollecting the many times over the last few years I've felt swallowed by the enormity of the implications of this research.

How do you put into words what happens when you come up against the system and find yourself surrounded and suffocated by ever-encroaching, shape-shifting brick walls? How do you put into words what happens when individuals collide with the system? Where does individual and collective responsibility begin? Where does it end?[17]

Perhaps scarpering away with my tail between my legs would've been the sensible thing to do. But before I came to my senses, I accepted a health charity's funding to understand the tobacco industry's marketing and business industry strategies in relation to e-cigarettes.[18]

There are still regular contradictory reports about whether e-cigarettes are "good" or "bad." A crude pro- or anti-e-cigarette split has been playing out in the media and peer-reviewed academic journals for several years, with researchers sometimes asked to "pick a side." To frame findings in a particular way, often guided by reviewers' personal views on the subject. To draw policy implications and wide-reaching conclusions from datasets and exploratory studies that can't offer such insights.

Behind closed doors and in Data Vaults, there are stories of conspiracy, coercion, fear, and powerlessness obscuring multiple truths and the public's comprehensive understanding of an issue central to their health and well-being. Truths, perhaps, that can be safely explored through creative analytical writing practices using verbatim quotes from multiple "traditional" data sources, including interview transcripts.

I sent myself off on a narrative non-fiction writing course for almost a week to try to make sense of my experiences of studying the controversial public health topic. On day 2, I had a revelation. I needed to write a (post)modern fable about scientific truth(s) (that would never see the light of day). Until now.

The day breaks through a bloated cloud. I stop to soak up the sunrise. It's surprisingly warming, even in my vapour-like state.

I wipe what would be greasy fingers to access my OneDrive. Somehow manage to type the words *Inside-the-Echo-Chamber*. My dated notes appear. They are excitable, digital scribbles. The beginning of a brainstorm.

It's the fifth of November 2017.

Modern fable

SILENT TRUTHS: *E-Cigarette Science and Fiction*
SILENT TRUTHS: *E-Cigarette Science and Some Fiction [or (Some) Fiction]*
SILENT TRUTHS: *E-Cigarette Sciencey Fiction (?)*

Tells the story of not being able to tell the story.

When your work is to investigate private sector involvement in public health, much of your work is neither public nor healthy.

A lot of silent truths remain untold for reasons that will (or may) never become apparent.

Your research makes you distrustful (maybe comes across to some as paranoid), fearful, has an impact on your mental and physical well-being, and leaves you feeling powerless. Helpless. You want to give up. And all these things help to maintain the status quo – prop up silent power structures that perpetuate. If we all gave up or were discredited, became too scared to speak out, burnt out, or got ill . . . what would happen? There would be no dissenting voices. There would only be silence.

A book about silent truths. My truth as I searched for and tried to tell the truth about e-cigarettes. The truth of others who told me their varying truths about e-cigarettes along the way. And a reflection of truth itself.

Why is this important? On the surface of it, statistics appear, policies are made, consensuses (is this even a word?) are reached. But there's a lot going on behind closed doors – silent truths – that is left untold. Why? Cock-up, conspiracy, coercion, fear, or a mixture of all?

It's 7 November 2017.

Hooray! I have the structure and chapter outline for **Inside the Echo Chamber**.[19]
Chapter 1 – Welcome to the circus
"Take notes. Take lots of notes. You have a ringside seat at the circus, and one day you're going to want to write about this" – words from a prophetic prof – [it's summer 2012] – OBSTACLES – prof's ideology – other profs' ideologies – too many ideologies – too many clashes – too many questions, not enough answers – how to predict what might happen in the future? – this is only the beginning . . .
Chapter 2 – The tobacco control wars
Quote – I'm a "narcissist" (a narcissist!) for studying e-cigarettes in this way [from someone who works in public health] – things are starting to get messy – OBSTACLES – before (during the tobacco wars) the tobacco industry was bad (it lied about killing people), public health was good – public health was united in a common enemy – now faction-fighting has begun – we publish a commentary calling for a unified tobacco-harm-reduction strategy (de Andrade and Hastings 2013) – divide and conquer . . . [it's May 2013]
Chapter 3 – Danger, danger
It's not even 10:00 a.m., and I'm being branded a murderer – OBSTACLES – anyone who's anti-e-cigs is being getting attacked by a powerful lobby that's starting to emerge (introduce the independents – "nascent interlopers") – I'm doing radio interviews after publishing in the BMJ (de Andrade, Hastings, and Angus 2013) – is the marketing of e-cigarettes tobacco marketing reinvented? – I'm being branded as the anti-e-cig public health expert – tell us, the media asks, are e-cigs a

good or bad thing? – this is missing the point and detrimental to public health – the devil is in the detail, but the detail is being obscured by a binary, black-and-white framing of the issue, I want to say, but that's quite a boring media debate – there is no debate without conflict – we get a letter from a company threatening some sort of legal action . . . [it's early 2014]

Chapter 4 – The Data Vault

"Just to be clear, you must never publish this data" [it's late 2017] – I'm on the phone, dealing with an urgent student matter, when the words hit my inbox. A familiar wave of dread washes through me – the shaking begins again – OBSTACLES – I went quiet – after the threats, I got scared, tired of it all, retreated – started focusing my energies on creative community engagement with marginalised communities (I'm dreaming of a research programme called Measuring Humanity these days) – I've started questioning, "What is evidence?" – [flash back to December 2015] – I get some courage again, put in another e-cig bid, this time to investigate e-cigarette business strategies – I get it, on the condition that I interview industry – elite interviews with tobacco executives = gold dust – incredible insights, but sensitive information – people are defaming each other left, right, and centre – analysis, peer review – lean heavily on "one side" – position yourself as pro- or anti-e-cig – defend, defend, defend – publish – now I'm not allowed to publish the data? – PANIC – "You can publish interpretations of the data" – oh? – scientific interpretivism?

Chapter 5 – Science vs. science fiction

My datasets are full of people slagging off the science – the same science used by different stakeholders, serving different (self-serving) purposes – it's tough to know what science to believe, difficult to distinguish science from science fiction – tobacco companies slagging off the science of other tobacco companies – public health experts slagging off the science of other public health experts – published, peer-reviewed science, now part of the evidence base, being cited and re-cited and accepted as scientific facts – knowledge and science being built on what some are calling "scandals" – these are informing policy decisions – OBSTACLES – how can I tell this story in a way that will protect me? Protect others? Protect my data? Protect the academy? Most of all, be truthful? What is truth? Why is everyone telling me a different story while telling me they're telling me the truth?

It's 9:05 a.m. in the real world, and I suddenly feel drained. The whole world is in some variation of lockdown, and to be honest, I don't know if the fantasy I'm enacting "in here" is more or less surreal than the reality "out there."

***

++ SARA M'S PIG MEMORY NOTES: APRIL 1, THE FUTURE – REFERRED BY VERITAS INC. – SECURITY ANALYSIS AND NETWORK INFORMATION TECHNOLOGY (SANITY) DIVISION ++

Presents as engaged. Animated even. Claims to know there's a truth out there that needs to be uncovered. She "can see it." She can see this "hyperreality" in her mind "so clearly." Claims everything is "connected." None of this is just happening. It's all carefully planned to perfection. Everything going on in my head, in your head, in every-one's head is controlled. But it's so subtle, so beautifully created that it's almost impos-sible to wrap your head around. Showing signs of severe delusion (see her Downloaded thoughts below). Suggest a fourteen-day Protective Order.

– Professor Ebba

1 April, 1900h

Row 7. Seat A. I'll never forget my seat allocation on the last-minute flight from Here to There for two reasons. One: I kept the ticket. Two: the view from 7A was incredible. Not out the window (it was dark by the time we'd boarded). But the view of 2C. Or at least it was for about twenty seconds, when time stood still.

Now, I don't believe in magic. I'm firmly grounded in reality. I know what is – and what is not – within the realms of possibility. So I can't begin to explain what happened to me when I saw that person standing there.

But I'll try.

Sam took my breath away.

They were one of the last to board, didn't seem bothered. Took their time fit-ting a leather laptop bag into the overhead compartment. From where I was sit-ting, they looked statuesque. Dark hair that wasn't curly, wasn't straight. Designer clothes as if they'd been stitched on to a chiselled body.

It was "a dis/orienting experience." I felt a complete "dis/jointedness of time and space," in touch with "entanglement of here and there, now and then." It was haunting even, "a ghostly sense of dis/continuity," a "quantum dis/continuity" (Barad 2010).[20]

I found myself drawn to them, wanting to sit and just *be with* them until some-one dragged me away, kicking and screaming.

Screaming.

The noise in my head. As our plane's nose sniffs the sky, I hastily order a white wine from the toothy air-attendant. Down it before she moves on. Order another.

I sip and stare into the abyss through the tiny window to my left. Definitely catching a glimpse of their elbow at one point. Let it go.

I have just over an hour to pull myself towards myself and mentally prepare myself for days ahead of me. Days of nothingness. Days of uncertainty. I have no idea where I'm going or why I'm going there, but I know I need to get away from fourteen days of prescribed torture in the form of a Protection Order.

I'm tired of everybody telling me they know what's best for me. I know what's best for me.

I've drained my emergency stash fund for this return trip, but it's worth it. I need to get away and think clearly. I'm onto something. Something colossal. On the cusp of something so ground-breaking that the rubble will never shift.

As my mind becomes anesthetised, I let it wander through the debris from the ground zero that will follow when my job here is done. I imagine what the little people will do when they discover that every single thing they've ever believed to be true is a lie. When they learn that the fights they've been having with "others" on virtual platforms to defend good causes, great people, are nothing more, nothing less than puppetry. Public spats with barbed words and shadowy pictures to right the wrongs of this world . . . nothing more, nothing less than role-playing.

Slaves fighting over who's going to be their next Master.

An almighty anarchy will follow, I imagine, as the minions rebel. As they stop Uploading, stop swiping, stop tagging, stop listening. Start thinking. And then what?

I hit a brick wall.

I just need time. Time to hoover up the seemingly disparate bytes scattered across the Sphere-Blue Drive. Time to ingest the digital, hermeneutic crumbs guiding me to the cannibalistic witch's house made of every consumable good known to mankind.

Time.

But time moves forward; it never moves back. [Rule # 1].

Just a few years ago, this flight would've taken just under four hours. Now fifty-five minutes in, the seat belt and body harness spontaneously strap itself around me as we nose-tumble to the ground. I stretch in my life-saving straightjacket, strain my neck to sneak a peek at 2C's cheek.

It happens again. My breath gets caught at the back of my throat, flutters in my stomach, which could be nerves or excitement.[21]

A booming voice blasts through the cabin, reminding us of our instructions under the Global Disembarkation Act. Eyes down, lips sealed, fingertips at the ready. Our life-saving restraints automatically release. At once, 349 pairs of eyeballs drop. We disembark two by two in an orderly fashion, much like mute, mismatched mammals. No one dares to speak as we swipe our digits across a flickering avatar, as we honour the Noble Silence, as we tag ourselves into this new land, as we Upload our new memories.

I hear their voice for the first time between beeps as we travelator through the lengthy security corridor.

"So what brings you to these shores?" They've somehow made it through the crowd to be by my side. I'm tickled pink with cheeks to match. This is not like me at all.

"A break . . . um . . . a . . . sort of escape." I never stutter.

Their eyes crinkle as they chuckle warmly.

"An escape, huh? I'm intrigued." Our marching turns to a meander as we enter the Holding Hub. I fiddle with the handle of my carry-on bag.

"It's complicated," I say. "I don't really want to get into it."

My cheeks change to fuchsia as a wave of molten lava floods my face. They sense my discomfort.

"I'm Sam." They reach out their right arm as if to shake hands. For a moment, it all disappears. The noise, the need to know, the nerves. I feel absolved from the shackles of my mind as we connect, hand to hand. Eye to eye.

"Sara."

"How do you feel about some company?" they ask. "Has your bag been tagged to your hotel?"

I mentally scroll through the contents of my carry-on. Toothbrush, next-generation device, toothpaste (one of the buy-one-get-one-free ones), charger, one-terabyte memory stick (x 17) (in a little, black pouch), black underwear (x 2), T-shirts (charcoal, x 2), a pair of jeans (black), a scarf (purple).

"Um . . . uh . . . this is my bag." Shuffling from heel to toe, I realise how little I've planned for my escape. I don't know where I'm going. I don't know where I'm staying. I haven't thought beyond this moment.

The plan is, the plan's going to change. [Rule #3]

Right here, right now, all I know is that I'm standing in front of a human with a touch of deity, with nothing but a carry-on and clothes I threw on about fifteen hours ago.

"No bag?"

"No bag."

"And you're going . . . ?"

"I have no idea where I'm going . . ."

The reality of my situation hits me like a tidal wave. I'm on the run. Again.

"I need to find the toilet."

"Okay. I'll be here . . . ?" I hear Sam say as I scurry away, my heart racing.

Where am I going? What am I doing? Is there anywhere to hide? Is there anywhere to hide from my thoughts?

In the cubicle, I splash some ice-cold water in my armpits. As the toilet disinfects itself, I search for the little black pouch in my carry-on. The one with the seventeen one-terabyte memory sticks. The one with my manual backup.

I start unpacking my bag like a person possessed. It definitely isn't hiding in the jeans or tees. The blood dancing in my cheeks just minutes ago drains. I start trembling. Aftershocks ripple through my body, getting caught at the base of my spine, where there's a throbbing now. I slide to the frozen floor, catching a glimpse of the white mask that is my face in the mirror.

I'm clutching my chest at the spot where there's meant to be an Emotion-Defibrillator ©.

Little black pouch. LITTLE BLACK POUCH! My mind is sprinting backwards along the travelator, at the swipe screen, in row 7, seat A. I would never have left my bag unattended, not even after two glasses of wine. It was sitting between my feet, annoying me and the air-attendant.

SO WHERE IS IT? WHERE IS THE LITTLE BLACK POUCH? The screaming, it's back.

SAM!

Ahhh. . .

This really isn't going according to plan.

The plan is,

the plan's going to change.

[Rule #3]

Jumbled.

"It's okay," I tell myself. "This is what happens when I panic. It'll pass. Everything passes. This isn't real."

But as I pick myself off the floor and repack the contents of my carry-on, I realise that this is real. The little black pouch is gone. So has thirty-four minutes.

Time moves forward; it never moves back. [Rule #1]

I'm mentally plotting my next move as I step out into the terminal. My heart skips another beat. Not too far in the distance, with their back to me, is Sam.

They're talking to a hyperactive synth, who appears to be waving her arms in an excitable act of malfunction. Her gesticulations grow wilder as I approach, her pitch more piercing yet imperceptible. Sam turns around, does a double take.

"Are you okay?" they ask.

"What do you mean?" I pout.

"You look really pale."

"Actually, there's been a bit of a situation." I bite my bottom lip.

"Sam, I've got to go. I've lost something important and need to retrace my steps. Enjoy the rest of your night." I turn away before they can spot the sadness in my eyes.

"Sara, wait. Is it this?"

Angels chant a virtuous anthem of doom in unison as a miracle appears in their hand – my little black pouch.

"But . . . how? How is this possible?" I'm gasping for breath again.

"You left it on the plane. The synth scanned herself into footage of us together on the travelator and came to find me."

I swoop in and unzip it.

One, two . . . five . . . eight. . .

. . . eleven. . .

. . . twelve, thirteen. . .

. . . sixteen. . .

And relax.

Seventeen mega memory sticks in my hand.

Sam's staring at me, eyes wide open. I can't tell if they're startled or amused.

"Are those memory sticks?" they ask. "Like the ones we used to use in the dark ages?"

"You mean the ones we used not so long ago," I correct them, "before the Cloud and Sphere-Blue Drive. It was just the other day, you know."

"Fine, I'll give you that. But why would anyone in their right mind still use them? You have to carry them around and . . ." They smile. "You clearly lose them."

"Sam," I say, "I carry them around so I don't lose my mind. There's a darkness that I'm carrying that's in desperate need of some light . . ."

I feel this strange and overwhelming need to keep talking, sharing with this stranger, connecting with this stranger. Being with this stranger. I want to be safe with this person in a place I don't think exists. A place where I can lie down and rest, where everything makes sense around me. A spot where the swirling stops. Where everyone speaks the truth. Where no one is out to hurt you.

Surely, I can't be feeling these feelings? There's no Emotion-Defibrillator © attached to my heart; this feeling can't be real,

I tell myself.

The electric shocks flooding from my heart through my chest are just those familiar terror tremors, nothing to be worried about here.

This is just pure terror at the thought of losing the actual truth, not some sort of synthetic pleasure pumping through my being,

I tell myself,

Nobody feels pleasure without help anymore,

I remind myself.

We just aren't capable anymore. It's suffering or nothing,

I remind myself.

Numbness or nothing.

"This isn't possible, Sam," I hear myself say. "I feel we've met before."

I'm standing here in a daze, trying to make sense of the maze connecting my mind and my middle.

Then a breezy bullet train trip and a short taxi ride to a Kava Bar known to locals as The Church. They enforce a strict no-booze policy. Just Kava on tap (and fizzy water if you're thirsty). No hangovers, no anxiety, no tense muscles, no interference with basic, brain-based skills. Pure intoxication without the stress. Borderline bliss, but too sedated to notice.

I hadn't been to a Kava Bar in years.

They're playing best hits from Behind the Noise.[22] "Complications" by källa[23] is blasting from the speakers when we saunter in.

"*Are we the comet in a clouded sky? Space travelling, just passing by. Are we the ghosts in a crowded room? They send the same certain doom . . .*"

"*Are you the camera that I hide behind? Just let me focus on what's in your mind. Am I the pebble stuck inside your shoe? We're both lost and don't know what to do . . .*"[24]

"Are you lost?" Sam asks me while ordering two cinnamon-flavoured Kava Cocktails. It's my favourite spice; it's almost like they can read my mind.

"*The compilations . . .,*" I say.

"What do you mean?" Their eyes zoom in on mine.

"'*I'll isolate myself, 'til there's no safety net . . .*'[25] The words of the song. I was there when they wrote it. I was Behind the Noise." I reach for one of the stemmed glasses that's just been gently placed in front of us.

"Cheers."

"Cheers."

We lock eyes. Swallow simultaneously.

I feel instantly lighter. It's amazing how holding a bit of blown glass can make you feel so sophisticated. I take another sip. Sink deeper into calmness.

Next thing I know, I'm sharing. Oversharing. Telling Sam about how I ended up in Beguile after bouncing around one community after another, trying to piece together the broken story of my childhood.

"Something magical happened when I found The Futile Forest and saw The Green Man. He was epic. Made from chunks of bark and stems and grass. Thinking about how he got there, how he found peace and became a Forest Guardian, how he stood for all the ancestors who came before him, made my problems shrink to the size of the mushrooms at his feet. And everyone who looked at him saw something different. That made me feel better too. Knowing that whatever I saw was what I saw. No need to beg for people to believe me. Best I've felt in forever."

"When did you feel your worst?" Sam asks.

"Fifteen years ago. My attempt to escape from the winter of doom."

Next thing I know, I'm word-vomiting some more. Telling them how I ran away from home like some cold-blooded chameleon. The one day I was convinced the people around me loved me; the next I felt like I was being given marching orders just as the Three Wise Men returned from another trip round the sun. I still don't understand why.

Sam's eyes are getting softer and softer, much like my biceps and triceps and calves and quads and . . .

"Should we take a seat on those bar stools?" I start floating there before my sentence stops. Sam stays at the bar to order another round.

I use the time to check my phone. There are a dozen messages or so from The Community. I'd just taken off; they're worried about me.

Another message flashes across my screen: "Hey sorry. I know its late. Call tmrw if its not 2 late. I thnk Im on to something x."

Numinous.[26]

I find it mildly irritating that he uses e-speak in messages, must remember to tell him to stop. After I call him. This sounds promising.

Sam navigates through circles of strangers who appear to be staring and smiling at us as if we're long-lost friends. Settles next to me on a chrome bar stool. Then the bustling stops. Everyone else disappears. They're definitely still there. Sucking on their vaporisers, sipping their sedatives in silence.

"I got us the Root Juice one this time." They narrow their enigmatic eyes as they pass me a deep-purple mixture of mystery. "Kava and Root Juice . . . surely a drink of darkness?" A penetrating look.

I flick my hair back. My floppy neck rolls back as I laugh. In my head, it's a wholehearted, deep belly laugh with gravitas and strength. In reality, I may be snorting.

"Nothing to worry about," I say, taking a swig. "Root Juice is magical. I had it on one of the Colony Camps."

Sam's eyes widen. "You've been on a Colony Camp? When?"

"Just before the Tipping Point. I was on one of the last flights out before the Global Disembarkation Act was passed." I try to get more comfortable on the bar stool.

"That's insane. I don't know anyone who's managed to get to the Camps. Well, I've heard rumours from the odd hack, but nothing to be taken too seriously. People will make anything up for attention. But you . . ." Sam stops for a generous sip. "You're being serious?"

"Yes. Deadly serious."

I feel powerful. As if I have insider knowledge. As if I'm important. As if I have another monumental secret. I don't usually talk about this truth and the feeling of helplessness it drags along with it, but right now in this Kava Bar, it's all I'm experiencing. I know something that others can only cobble together from fragmented news clips or e-Learning platforms. And that's only part of the story. With knowledge comes power. And responsibility.

"It must've been terrifying," Sam eventually says. "The natives . . . how scary are they?"

I'm trying to swallow, but those words send a jolt through my body. Kava Root Juice shoots right up my nose. In one second, I'm high as a kite, my mind giddily somersaulting through abandoned memory archives.

"Between you and me," I lean in and whisper, "the natives aren't scary at all. They're alive. They feel things. I've never come across so much happiness and warmth even though they have nothing to their name. I'm in awe of them." I down the rest of my Juice.

I'm not sure how to read Sam, who's staring at me as if I'm certifiable. Someone who sits on the cusp of madness. Someone who dances in the shadows.

Then Sam's looking left, right, and left again. Scanning the bar. "You know, this kind of chat could get you into trouble," they whisper in my ear. I feel their breath on my neck. "If I were you, I'd keep quiet."

It isn't a threat, but I feel the need to stop talking.

I reach for my mobile and scan through messages. I'm wondering what Numinous means about being on to something when Sam takes the phone out of my hand and presses the touchscreen with their right forefinger.

"What are you doing?"

"Just trying to make your battery run out. Come on." They smile. "Don't let technology ruin this experience. Let's turn your phone off."

Sam does exactly that without waiting for permission.

At this moment, we both know we're relaxing into a force much greater than us.

Something is happening.

We get up to leave. It's almost 1:00 a.m.

"Where should we go?" Sam asks as we drift to the door.

"Anywhere." The cool air caresses us. "We're scripting this." [Rule #4]

***

INTERLUDE – BLURRING THE RESEARCHER, THE RESEARCHED, AND THE RESEARCH

Who's scripting this? I wonder.

Is it me, Marisa de Andrade, at 5:24 a.m. on the nineteenth of December 2021, not long after the passing of the Cold Moon at 11:32 p.m., the longest full moon of the year?

Is it me, Marisa, author of a book introducing post-qualitative inquiry, humanities, and arts-informed methodologies and theories to public health researchers?

An author who, like clockwork or by magic, gets a surge of energy and creativity each lunar cycle?

Am I writing this as we, in the UK, retreat into what's fast looking like another enforced hibernation?

Or is Sam scripting this at another time, in another place? Sam, who's appeared rather suddenly in Sara's life with some uncanny connection to her. Sam, who knows so much about Sara without knowing Sara at all.

Or is In-Credible the author? The somewhat-audacious researcher who we've left on a rooftop in Beguile, *experiencing* her data *with* Community Members rather than analysing it from behind her computer screen, where she's meant to be.

Who's scripting this?

These fictional characters created to tell the stories of the "real" humans I met during my fieldwork, whose stories I can only tell through anonymised vignettes?[27]

Or those "real" humans finding a place within those imaginary ones? Within myself as I relate to them and to my data as I try to make meaning of it?

Who's scripting this?

As I ask this question over and over in the stillness of the pre-sunset morning, I sense all these humans – the "real" and imaginary – settle beside me and within me like apparitions. This feels like a "ghostly matter," a "haunting" of the "sociological imagination." I float towards Avery F. Gordon's belief that "to be haunted, is to be tied to historical and social effects . . . to attend to such queer effects . . . to negotiate the relationship between what we only see and what we know" (Gordon and Radway 2008).[28]

I can feel what Avery means when she says that "haunting is a mediation," "a process that links an institution and an individual, a social structure and a subject, and history and a biography." I agree that, through her writing, "she restores to social theory that attentiveness to the textures and meanings of experience that was bracketed off at the moment the sciences embraced the quantitative and conceded the province of the qualitative and the imaginary to literature and the arts" (Gordon and Radway 2008).[29]

What if the opposing paradigms could co-exist, side by side, informing each other? Breathing life into each other's meanings and positionalities?

Speaking different academic languages, yes, but what if they could be in conversation rather than knocking heads? Respectfully *affected* by one another?

I think public health scholars would certainly be open to this, perhaps claiming this is what the discipline's done all along as it navigated "the well-rehearsed qualitative/quantitative divide" (Blackman 2007).[30] A qualitative arm with clear limitations when it comes to sampling, generalising, drawing conclusions for policy and practice – though useful in informing a quantitative arm that tells us what's really going on – at scale.

But for this reductive qual-quant relationship to produce truly meaningful insights for those being "researched" – for the relationship to be healthy rather than dysfunctional – we need to pay attention to its underpinning foundations. Pay attention to the realities, ideologies, emotions, and inner worlds of the "researched," researchers – as well as the funders, journals, and institutions they're connected to – and how these attributes seep into each encounter and dataset.

The conundrum for public health is, *How?* How are we supposed to do this, methodologically? As Blackman puts it: "The challenge of developing post-positivist methods to do justice to the challenges that are raised, open up the question of what might count as 'empirical' within studies of affect." Quoting Barad, she puts forward the notion of "hauntology" as:

> [A] *"diffractive reading" (a term she [Barad] borrows from Donna Haraway), so that the displaced event or narrative can be interfered with. She terms this "diffraction as method" (Barad 2010),[31] in which texts, events, actors, and agencies are read "intra-actively" through one another. The use of the term intra-action, rather than "interaction," signals that texts are not separate and then brought together, but rather that texts (or statements, events, actors, and agencies) are always-already entangled in complex ways in practices. (Blackman 2007)[32]*

de Andrade quoting Blackman, who's quoting Barad, who's drawing from Haraway.

Who's scripting this?

Through physicist-philosopher Karen Barad's "ethico-onto-epistem-ology" framework, we all are. All of us – co-creating the haunted, magical worlds co-constructed by my characters, informed by my "participants" and other "human and non-human beings – are intra-actively co-constituting the world. Our entanglements make it impossible to separate ethics from ontology and epistemology when producing (scientific) knowledge through scientific practices" (Barad 2007).[33]

This quote takes me back to a lively exchange in my Humanities and Arts-Informed Methodologies in the Social Sciences postgraduate class a couple of months ago. We'd been reflecting on the nature of reality (ontology) as the groundwork to approaching research questions and how public health hardly ever "goes there."

Why would public health scholars need to position their work ontologically when there's an a priori assumption that the science-data-evidence informing the discipline is firmly grounded in an acceptable version of "reality"?

This makes it easier – necessary perhaps – to dismiss the science-data-evidence offered by the likes of shamans or druids or any other spiritual healers in touch with the dead or the land as hocus-pocus. After all, they interpret reality in a very different way from "others" around them – the definition of psychosis.

There's a lot of research concluding that it is impossible to distinguish between mystical or magical experiences and psychosis through phenomenological description – concerning the science of phenomena as separate to the nature of being – alone (Mitchell 2010). So to make sense of these psychotic phenomena, we need to understand how these experiences are "implanted" into the beliefs, ideals, and ethics of the person.[34] We need to know how the person *is in relationship with* so-called delusional beliefs.

"What I find astonishing when I'm doing fieldwork," I tell my class, "is how an individual and community's beliefs are inextricably linked to their experience of reality – and also their well-being. If they believe they'll be healed through chanting and a drumming circle or when speaking to their ancestors through Forest Guardians like The Green Man, then they are. They arrive feeling anxious, lost, alone, or depressed. They leave feeling connected, loved, heard, and well. Or at least better. It's astonishing, the power of the mind."

I pause to think about how this compares to the placebo effect in clinical settings when a PhD student says exactly that.

"Yes, it's like the placebo effect . . ."

Our minds meet in the same place. The cornerstone of scientific research is based on the notion of an "implant" (if you will) being "put in to" participants on clinical trials to test for drug efficacy. An inactive – some would say lazy – (non) drug is given to some people on the trial without their knowledge, while others get the "real" drug that's meant to "fix" them in some way, without their knowledge.

Clinical measurement, which is meant to capture both the safety and efficacy of the real (not pretend) drug, is achieved through a comparison of how both groups react. If participants' reactions are the same, regardless of whether they're on the real or imagined drug – and regardless of whether there's an improvement or not – science says the drug doesn't work.

What we don't talk about as much as we should is that most drugs on clinical trials don't pass this test. They can't eclipse the placebo effect – the power of the mind. Science journalist Eric Vance conceptualises this as the "theatre of medicine." Stories have power – superpowers – to heal. We feel better by the things we believe in. More so than the effectiveness of some drugs we are given (Vance 2016).

Through this framing, a "psychotic episode" in all its magical reality and splendour is a very effective pill. Even if that pill is a pine marten. Or a poem.

I want to keep telling my class about the nocebo, which, through the same logic, has a detrimental effect on well-being by expecting the worst from a treatment or diagnosis (welcome to the world of fear), but I'm running out of time. We still have a few formative assessments to get through the day.

We ease into the next group presentation on *Psychosis: Narrative Psychiatry as an Assets-Based Model* – a recorded Zoom and PowerPoint conversation between four students (three in the human form [via video]; the other there in spirit but unable to be there in the flesh [albeit it captured in film format]) (Yue et al. 2021).

As the technology settles, I think about Bruner's proposition that a story "operates as an instrument of mind in the construction of reality"(Bruner 1991).[35] How do we know what we know? And how do we make sense of that knowing through communication, not always written or verbal?

The recording starts, and I'm instantly aware that my students' thoughts appear to echo my thoughts. I haven't been going on about different interpretations of psychosis all that much in class, but they've appeared to latch on to some of the things I've said about the biomedical model being based on deficiency and pathological perspectives. That said, they aren't quoting me – they're critically analysing a book chapter in *Healing the Mind Through the Power of Story: The Promise of Narrative Psychiatry* (Mehl-Madrona 2010).

I haven't read this text.

The four thinkers reflect on how the National Health Service (NHS) defines *psychosis* as a disconnection from reality.

"And yet," Leandro asks, "who defines this reality? Is it fixed? Is it out there? Is it moving? Is it between us? Is it in my head? Or in our heads? Reality. Is it fluid? Relational or static?"

He goes on to wonder if symptoms are necessarily scary, negative, or a problem?

These are thoughts I've said out loud and heard from the "mentally unwell" I've encountered in my fieldwork.

Vennus continues by suggesting that we need to take seriously the ontology and epistemology of the individual experiencing psychosis instead of denying their experience as simply "mad." Drawing from the asset-based community development literature and narrative psychiatry, the suggestion is to move from the individual to the community with a focus on inclusivity: "Relational ontology engages with the processual. Life is interconnected, relational. This is more-than just multiple realities."

I think about Sara, The Community, and what they have that is so much more than the sum of their parts. So much more than their case notes, medical records, and diagnoses. They are relating creatively. Their experiences are creative-relational – a "dynamic conceptual frame for vibrant incisive research" that Jonathan Wyatt turned into the Centre for Creative-Relational Inquiry (CCRI):

> *CCRI fosters innovative qualitative research that places the relational at its heart and is situated, positioned, context-sensitive, personal, experience-near, and embodied; embraces the performative and the aesthetic; engages with the political, the social, and the ethical; problematizes agency, autonomy, and representation; cherishes its relationship with theory, creating concepts as it goes; is dialogical and collaborative; and is explicit and curious about the inquiry process itself. Creative-relational inquiry might include: detailed, close-up explorations of, for example, therapeutic and pedagogical relationships; the use of the arts and performance as a methodological approach; inquiries that put concepts and theories to work; and research that engages practitioners and the wider public – creatively, relationally – in and with such research.*[36]

We – Jonathan and I and the other associate directors, Rosie, Fiona, and Nini, along with others in the centre – have been playing with, plugging in, and putting creative-relational inquiry to work since its conception. This book is a product of creative-relational inquiry in action. It's troubling traditional approaches to researching public health, noticing how the topics we seek "answers for" in the discipline are in constant movement – not "fixed" in the reality of an individual, but situated within a wider social "relational reality."

This is the point Leandro is now making. Citing Rosiek, Snyder, and Pratt (2020), he notes, "Knowledge is co-created in relationships. Subjectivity and inter-subjectivity is valued. It embraces transformation, not only focuses on the ways of knowing, but also the ways of being, feeling, committing and living in the world."

The word *transformation* always riles me. It suggests that change – "real," genuine change – is possible for the most unequal in our world. That by researching disadvantaged communities – even through participatory, bottom-up approaches like in Measuring Humanity, where each Community Member is meant to be an equal and active participant in the process – life will somehow get better for The Community.

I'm not convinced the "reality" of pervasive structural inequalities allows for that to "truly" happen. We need systemic change. But I do believe that by using these creative-relational approaches to question what we know and how we know it, there is real opportunity to challenge public health research design, thereby challenging the findings they produce.

Why can't post-qualitative public health studies sit alongside clinical studies to inform research, policy, and practice when they're telling us something about the experience of health that positivist findings never will?

Emily, one of the other PhD students in the group, sums it up nicely:

> There is something powerful about the process of thinking with you about psychosis, about thinking with others. . . . Perhaps this has been an act of resistance – a small one, performing what we are advocating for – processes, relational. That something really happens in the act of engagement that is worth putting across.

I agree. These four scholars in a virtual space and in the flesh in class are performing "Slow Tiny Acts of Resistance (STARs)" (Harré et al. 2017),[37] much like the CCRI directors did when penning our journal special issues on qualitative inquiry as "activism in the academy (academic work, academic cultures, academic practices, etc.)" and "activism in the processes of research itself and activism beyond the academy, in the world" (Rodríguez-Dorans et al. 2021), "the act of collaborative research and writing opens up movement of thought – the rupture – the escape from the already known, however small and inconsequential each escape may seem to be" (Gale and Wyatt 2018; Speedy 2015).

I think about my collaborative researchers Sara and Sam. And In-Credible. And the new arrival, Numinous. I wonder what they would say at this point. What escape from the already known might they have to offer?

***

++ SARA M'S PIG MEMORY NOTES: APRIL 1, THE FUTURE – REFERRED BY VERITAS INC. – SECURITY ANALYSIS AND NETWORK INFORMATION TECHNOLOGY (SANITY) DIVISION ++

DOWNLOADED THOUGHTS CONTINUED – PROFESSOR EBBA

2 April, 1005h

I wake up to the sun in my eyes, its rays on my cheeks. The blackout curtains wide open, I stretch to inspect the scenery from high, high up.

Where am I?

Concrete.

And cement.

Cement and concrete.

Brutalist is back in fashion.

I'm in what appears to be a hotel room. A minimalist, upmarket one. White, black, chrome.

My carry-on luggage lies open on the thick grey carpet beside a single bed, its contents spread out as if part of a treasure trail.

My phone's plugged into one of the many sockets on the white wall in front of me, next to a rather-large flat-screen.

I feel as if I've had the best sleep in decades.

I'm alone.

I get out of bed, amazed by the definite spring in my step. I feel good.

I grab my phone, now fully charged, and turn it on while I inspect the room for a coffee machine or at least a kettle. No such luck.

As soon as the fingerprint on my right forefinger unlocks my phone, the screen starts flashing like a silent disco. Fourteen missed calls. Two messages. All from Numinous.

1:30 a.m.: "CALL ME XXX."

It isn't like him to shout in messages and send me three forceful kisses.

3:25 a.m.

"Sara – call me! Looks lke sum1s hacked in2 the Wlled Gdn x."

The Walled Garden. This could be serious.

I look around the room again, taking in all its angular features. A giant Anglepoise floor lamp peeking at me from above. A black-and-white Sputnik ceiling light with twelve perfect orbits.

It's so, so quiet. I'm alone, I realise again, this time taking in reality more fully. I've run away, again, to be safe and alone, again. My life alone.

I hit Numinous's number.

"Hi, Sara."

"The Walled Garden? What's going on?"

He starts laughing. "Hi, Sara. I'm okay, thanks. How are you?" More laughter.

"Stop messing around, Numinous. This could be serious. What's going on?"

"Nothing anymore. Everything's under control now, I think," he says.

"What do you mean everything's under control? You can't scare me like this, Numinous. Do you think this is funny?"

He clears his throat. "Not at all. Sorry. I didn't mean to make light of this. I thought there was a hack wandering through your Walled Garden, but looks like it was just a glitch. Everything's back to normal, not even a trace of malfunction. It's like it never happened. Maybe I was seeing things. I haven't slept in days . . . been following that other lead . . . I think I'm on to something . . ."

"So what do you think you're on to?" I start packing my things in my carry-on as if I have somewhere to go.

"I'm not sure exactly," Numinous says. "It's so subtle . . . almost imperceptible . . . but every now and then a code changes. Then it changes back. Like a flicker. You see it, then it's gone."

"A bit like The Walled Garden thing you thought you saw last night?"

"Hmmm . . . sort of. Except last night I thought there was some DPS going on."

"Meaning?" Numinous gets all techy when he gets excited or anxious or both. He knows I don't understand half of his white-hat hacking lingo.

"Meaning, I thought an application was running to capture data packets."

"Meaning?"

"Meaning, technically someone could see your data."

I freeze.

"Sara . . . Sara are you there?"

"Yes, I'm here. I can't really deal with this right now." I head towards the bathroom, my head suddenly spinning. "You sure everything's under control now?"

"I know. That's why I was trying to get hold of you. But I spent the rest of the night trying to trace it, and there's nothing there. I guess I can't say for sure, but I've tried every trick in the book. It's all clean."

"Okay," I say, turning on the shower.

"Where are you, anyway?"

"I can't tell you, Numinous. Just don't ask me these kinds of questions." The mirror starts steaming up. "Look, I've got to go."

"Okay, fine," he says. "Sara, just be careful, okay?"

"Always. I was born to be on the run." I hang up. Set my phone next to the basin. Step under the scalding water, where I feel right at home.

My mind races as I foam up.

Too much information to process.

Too short a space of time.

We're such badly built machines, I catch myself thinking.

We humans.

We think we're so smart and sophisticated, but we're full of

flaws. Layer

upon layer

upon layer

of unprocessed thoughts and memories and nightmares.

And dreams.

All just accumulating.   Amounting to nothing.

I turn off the tap.

I walk back into the bedroom, open my carry-on again, put on my charcoal T-shirt and black jeans.

I need to get out of here.

Moments later, I'm following a sign pointing to the Blossom Market in the Channel. I'm desperate for a coffee now and aware of a wave of anxiety crashing at my fingertips. They start playing a speedy tune on an invisible piano.

I pick up my pace until I'm surrounded by Channels that appear to have surfaced out of nowhere. As if someone's stuck them in my path. So cleverly generated it's difficult to believe they're basically cardboard cut-outs.

"Looks just like a City in Europe, doesn't it?" a voice says from behind me.

I turn around to face someone who looks vaguely familiar.

"Do I know you?" I feel as if I know this person.

"Sam," they say. We lock eyes for a moment. There's an instant relief. Then Sam looks away and drinks in the Channels. "It's just like the real deal."

"It is unreal," I marvel.

Silence.

"It's a beautiful day for exploring. How about we start walking and see where we end up?"

Sam points into the distance. I look beyond their fingertips. Nothing but blue skies and a ball of fire.

I think about what else I could be doing. Should be doing. About the reason I've run away again. Of the words I told Professor Ebba when she tried to get me to up my prescription.

Things have been speeding up since they were slowed down by Veritas Inc. You know that. I know that. We're going faster and faster, and I'm trying to make sense of it all. Not just for me, not just for The Community. For everyone. There's a lot of work to be done, and I don't want to be numbed out.

I'm almost there,

I remind myself.

Just need a bit more time to piece it all together,

I remind myself.

I ignore the wave of nausea crashing at my throat. The thought of sticking myself in a hotel room and figuring this all out alone threatens another swell.

"Sure," I say before I can change my mind. Spontaneously. As if I have no say in the matter. As if I'm surrendering to the possibility of peace for just one day. As if I really, really know Sam.

Next thing I know, we're walking along the waterway with the sun smiling down on us. I've forgotten I need caffeine.

Sam has a map in hand, but neither of us is paying much attention to directions. We're just drifting. Getting lost, then found, then lost again.

We stop to admire a pile of oversized bricks made to look like an abandoned old ruin. I follow Sam's gaze to a rustic sign painted green and orange: "MYSTIC MELONS." The Y a smiley face; the O a melon.

We exchange curious looks. Shrug our shoulders simultaneously. We're drawn towards the sign like snakes to an Arabic tune flowing from a flute in Aladdin. Enter the wooden space, half shop, half gallery. I've never seen a place like it.

"Mystic Medicine for the Modern Mind," another handwritten sign reads, just above a locked glass cabinet displaying mind-altering substances skilfully categorised and rated on a truth-thruthier-thruthiest ratio. There's one to remedy every human ailment with a promise to energise, equalise, elate, or quite simply blow your mind with truthiness.

Like kids in a dodo museum, we "Ooh" and "Aah" at each extinct pill or potion. The man behind the counter – crinkled in the face, dreadlocked in the hair, impossible to age – chuckles as we ogle.

"It was a different time," he says. "A time when people from here and people from the Colony Camps were mixed together . . . and when you took one of those" – he points at the cabinet – "everyone was the same." His eyes drift off to an unknown place. His face softens. "Actually, before you took one of those . . . everyone was the same." He nods knowingly into the unknown. "It was the beginning of the end." He's lost in his mind.

I sense a sadness. A second passes. It's replaced with mischief. He pulls a set of rusty keys from his pocket, lifts a small wooden box encrusted with dented silver and violet rocks from under the counter. Unlocks it. Gently removes what looks like two mints the size and colour of baby goldfish. He cups his left hand to create a pond for them.

"What are they?" Sam asks.

"Truth Bombs."

We zoom in to get a closer look. They remind me of the time I saw the sun rising over the Sahara, bursting with orange and the promise of a new beginning.

"Wow," I say. "They have a life of their own."

The man behind the counter chuckles again. "They sure do. Just one life . . . it's up to them to decide what to do with it."

I wonder if he's some pseudo-philosopher getting his kicks out of tricking strangers. Spouting existential nonsense at wanderers. Declaring metaphysical drivel to whoever happens to be passing by. I'm getting good vibes from him, though, so decide to call him the Oracle Man.

He looks me in the eyes. Turns to Sam. Smiles. "They're yours," he says.

Sam looks at him suspiciously. "Mine?"

"Well . . . you can share." Oracle Man turns to me. Smiles.

Sam's phone rings. "Excuse me, I have to take this."

"Hello . . . ?" There's a frown on Sam's face as they walk out the gallery.

I'm left standing at the counter, staring at the Truth Bombs. They look like they've changed colour now. As if the sun's slowly moved across the desert and bronze has made way for a sandy brown. I'm drawn to them like a camel to an oasis.

Before I know what's happening, I have one in my hand, between my lips. An explosion of syrupy melon. I close my eyes. Bliss.

When I open them again, Oracle Man is shining. Sam is standing beside me, looking panicked.

"What are you doing?"

One more Truth Bomb swims in Oracle Man's hand. He looks at Sam encouragingly.

Sam looks stunned. "Are you feeling alright?"

I'm finding the frightened-rabbit look on his face a little amusing, but other than that, I'm feeling just fine.

"I'm feeling just fine," I say. "Just do it. What are you so scared of, anyway?"

Fear flickers on Sam's face, then passes like a lifting fog. "Nothing. I'm not scared of anything." They shove the Truth Bomb in their mouth with a fierce intensity.

"Enjoy your journey into truth," Oracle Man says as we drift out the door.

"The truth only matters when it can be proven. There are wider forces at play,"[38] I hear myself saying as we follow the sun.

***

INTERLUDE – A DEEP DIVE INTO THE VALIDITY OF IMAGINATIVE TRUTH-TELLING

The truth.

Everyone I've met in my research has told me they're telling me the truth. When some truths contradict the truths of others, whose truth matters? And why does it keep changing?

A quote from *The Museum of Extraordinary Things*, written by the magical realist Alice Hoffman, springs to mind: "*The truth frightens people because it isn't stable. It shifts every day*" (Hoffman 2014).

It's 11:23 a.m. on 19 December 2021. Pandemic life is shifting every day. As Covid-19 continues to spread fear as fast as it's spreading disease, my mind drifts back to my abandoned modern fable *Inside the Echo Chambers*.

I think about other stories in public health that aren't making news headlines at this time. I think about stories that may be being silenced by dominant narratives coupled with the fear of pushing against the boundaries of propagating power structures. As feminist author Marilyn Frye puts it, "the powerful normally determine what is said and what is sayable . . . When the powerful label something or dub it or baptize it, the thing becomes what they call it" (Frye 1983).[39]

How might an imaginative exploration of truth-telling, and truth itself, unfold? And how would it be "useful" to public health?

It would certainly add to debates relating to the validity and value of fiction specifically, and humanities and arts-based methodologies more broadly, as research (Wyatt 2007; Crawford et al. 2015). It might also call into question the objectivity of science and process of policy formation through a creative-relational analysis unravelling multiple contradicting subjectivities and complexities of power (Raimondi, Moreira, and de Barros 2020). It could add further weight to the argument that personal and experience-near research needs to be accepted as evidence alongside positivist approaches in public health research, policy, and practice (Rodríguez-Dorans et al. 2021; Wyatt 2018).

With some of the world in some kind of lockdown (again) due to a communicable disease, I'm reminded (again) of my research on non-communicable disease. I see a similar story of power and fear playing out in the media, social media, academy, and policy circles. And I'm thinking (again) about putting "theory into action through storytelling" to explore how "knowing and being . . . is not about creating stable, coherent, finished, and identifiable knowledges but instead focuses on engaging with the world as shifting, partial, unfinished, and animated by feeling and imagination" (Holman Jones 2018).[40]

I reflect on Vera Caine and colleagues' exploration of the functions of fictionalization in narrative inquiry. "Fictionalizing," they say, "has become a common and often unquestioned part of responding to concerns about anonymity raised by research ethics boards" (Caine et al. 2016).

While this may be the case for boards overseeing the arts, humanities, and some approaches to social science, this has not been my experience of public health research, particularly in tobacco control. Leaning firmly on the medical model and epistemological positioning of objective truth (Berwick 2005), fictionalising in this realm is largely considered to be aligned with mistruth.

I remember trying to publish an article on the emotional entanglements in public health research, particularly e-cigarettes, with a group of (then) early-career researchers. We considered the use of fiction to protect identities of participants and create distance between ourselves and our experiences. One colleague noted that "it sounds too much like we are making stuff up."

The lead author went on to use semi-fictionalised vignettes to synthesize shared, salient experiences while preserving anonymity in a commentary exploring how early-career public health researchers, studying e-cigarettes in particular, are "caught in the middle" of "complicated moral and affective landscapes" with "personal drivers and emotive feeling" shaping policy and research agendas (Lucherini 2018).[41] These vignettes, though just one paragraph each and embedded within a conventionally approached and structured article, were a tentative foray into the creative-relational approaches that I think public health needs to embrace (or at least gently cuddle).

But how to use creative (non)fiction without being accused of fabrication, and why use it in the first place? I use it as a methodology here as other alternatives aren't available. Tobacco control is a relatively small field, tobacco harm reduction smaller still. The e-cigarette research domain in particular is minute if you're an insider. Dominant voices on either side of the e-cigarette "camp" pop up repeatedly with similar arguments. There are only a handful of key multinationals with a stake in the market. Their products and business strategies are unique and easily distinguishable if you pay attention to detail. And these people and companies are powerful. They have financial and legal clout and/or influential positions in the academy and/or are authoritative figures in policy and media circles. Put simply, you don't mess with them.

Writing about these experiences is *not* about exposing any person, company, organisation, or institution. This inquiry is *not* part of the blame game – it does not accuse any entity or anyone of wrongdoing. It simply attempts to creatively unravel the complexities of seeking and telling the "truth" about e-cigarettes – a controversial and contested area of research – from multiple perspectives with competing "truths." Anonymity and pseudonymisation weren't an option. I tried that, coded data to obscurity, and even still it was blindingly obvious (at least to me and, I suspect, those in the field) who the participants were based on strong views.

I was then faced with another challenge when collecting, analysing, and finally publishing data from this dataset. Interpreting data, on this topic, appeared to rely on adopting a particular ideological position. When we attempted to adopt an "ideological blanksheet," impassioned reviewers suggested we hadn't considered the other side of the story. There wasn't enough or too much criticism of industry and tobacco harm reduction.

The need to tell the nuanced story became increasingly apparent as I realised that the e-cigarette narrative being framed as "good" or "bad" may be the real detriment to public health. It shuts down important debates, research questions, and findings. By presenting this as a black-or-white issue, we lose the grey, which is where some of the clues are about what's really going on.

My first problem was how to "co-compose" – to introduce the voice of myself as researcher and also participants (for example, tobacco industry executives) without being accused of reinforcing industry narratives. My second was how to portray this negotiation when public health journals typically ask research-ers to report findings objectively with clear conclusions and policy implications. Both were near-impossible tasks using quantitative or qualitative methodologi-cal approaches deemed to be "acceptable" or "valid" in high-quality, "credible" public health journals.

So I thought about how our data, derived from two key studies on e-cigarettes using a triangulated analysis of traditional methods of data collection, could be used creatively. How could twenty-eight elite interviews with the tobacco industry and other stakeholders; 1,022 company reports, investor analyses, press releases, and government consultation responses; and 991 media reports, images, social media posts, and advertisements be used to tell a different story?

I assumed the position of "situated speaker" engaged in "knowing/telling" something about this research as I "perceive[d] it." I didn't "try to play God" – presenting evidence as one of those "disembodied omniscient narrators claiming universal and atemporal general knowledge" (Denzin and Lincoln 2005).[42]

Consider this writing as a form of inquiry "validated as a method of knowing" in the "political/social world we inhabit – a world of uncertainty" (Denzin and Lincoln 2005).[43] It wedges an opening in dominant public health paradigms and invites you in to explore the complexities and perplexities of the system we're all in and relating to (Ellis and Bochner 1996).

Situated within a spacious post-modernist environment of doubt, there is a compulsion to know how I claim to know – how do I locate myself as "knower" and "teller"? Without the need to conform to a framework, I can step outside of predictable (social) scientific writing, allowing reflexivity of research – past, present, or future. Without the pressure of "getting it right," I can only get "it differently contoured and nuanced" (Denzin and Lincoln 2005).[44]

Triangulation, triumphed as validation in qualitative methods, makes way for crystallisation as there are more than three ways to view the world. How you see it depends on your "angle of repose" (Denzin and Lincoln 2005).[45]

So where will my story start?

I need an imaginative entry point into this creative-nonfictional representation of "reality." My mind immediately flits to George Orwell's *Animal Farm* (Orwell 1945), so I found myself web-searching for its plot summary. I like this one:

> *Animal Farm is a novel about a group of animals who take control of the farm they live on. The animals get fed up of their master, Farmer Jones, so they kick him out. Once they are free of the tyrant Jones, life on the farm is good for a while and there is hope for a happier future of less work, better education and more food. However, trouble brews as the pigs, Napoleon and Snowball, fight for the hearts and minds of the other animals on the farm. Napoleon seizes power by force and ends up exploiting the animals just as Farmer Jones had done. The novel ends with*

the pigs behaving and even dressing like the humans the animals tried to get rid of in the first place.[46]

These pigs have power.

Pork Power.

I think I'll enter my imaginary world through a story called "Pork Power."

***

++ SARA M'S PIG MEMORY NOTES: APRIL 2, THE FUTURE – REFERRED BY VERITAS INC. – SECURITY ANALYSIS AND NETWORK INFORMATION TECHNOLOGY (SANITY) DIVISION ++

DOWNLOADED THOUGHTS CONTINUED – PROFESSOR EBBA

2 April, 1307h

"Enjoy your journey into truth," Oracle Man says as we drift out the door.

"The truth only matters when it can be proven. There are wider forces at play,"[47] I hear myself saying as we follow the sun.

We settle in the nearest sunniest spot, two chairs in an outdoor café on an unnamed square where a few people are sipping seriously small coffees, pretending to be European. I remember I wanted one earlier, but my desire for caffeine is now non-existent. There's a smell of smoked sausages from an open grill nearby, but it does nothing for me. I've lost my appetite. All I can see, sense, and feel is Sam.

It's the same feeling as yesterday at the airport, but more intense.

Connected.

I can feel Sam feels it too.

We bask and beam for what feels like eternity without needing to say a word.[48]

Then I speak. "Do you think our 'chance' meeting is fate?"

"I missed my flight yesterday." Sam lies back in a metallic chair with closed eyes. "I was meant to be on an earlier plane but got stuck in traffic . . ."

My body melts into my metallic chair. I close my eyes.

"Maybe the stars were aligned. . .," Sam says, eyes still closed.

A surge of gratitude overwhelms me, pours from a place somewhere in my chest, rushes through my gut to my toes, shoots back up my body through my spine, makes my head tingle.

I haven't *felt* in forever, but I instinctively know this is what gratitude feels like. I'm one with this moment. There are no other moments. There is no other way this moment should be. This moment is perfect. I want to reach out and touch the moment – thank the moment for being this moment. But then the moment disappears.

"Thank you, universe." The words flow out of me as if they have a life of their own. My eyes are still closed. I feel so peaceful.

In my mind, I'm in a soundproof recording studio. There's a mixing desk, a few microphones and amplifiers, and some other analogue and digital equipment. I'm the only one there. This is a safe place.

A steady vibration whirrs in the background, a distortion of sort, but it isn't disturbing me.[49] It's grounding me. Leading me to what's Behind the Noise.[50]

I lean in to the buzzing until there's a stillness, then I reach for a blank sheet of paper and pen positioned right next to the Volume button.

This page becomes "a material stage for creative activity" that flows through me in the form of words and musical notes.[51] As the music bursts from me like a river against a saturated bank, I start remembering things I'd forgotten. Accessing memories I didn't know I had – some soothing, others terrifying – but the music holds me and releases me simultaneously.[52]

> *"You haven't seen this side of me.*
> *Find a way to set you free.*
> *Bruised and battered and bleeding bad.*
> *And these three things don't make me sad.*
> *I want to leave you left for dead.*
> *It won't be what you expected, it won't be what you expected . . ."*
> *"It won't be what you expected, it won't be what you expected . . ."*[53]

With a sudden jolt, I'm back in the square. That was Sam's voice.

"Great song," Sam says, "and I love the artwork on the poster."

I see it in my mind too. A penny in chains. A penny behind bars. "A Penny Vacant."[54]

How? How does Sam know these things? It's almost as if they can read my mind. Sam gently opens their eyes as if waking up from a lifetime of sleep.

"You're Behind the Noise too?" I ask quietly.

The Truth Bombs,

    I tell myself.

Must be the Truth Bombs.

We're holding each other in our gazes. Sam doesn't have to say a word.

"I'm not sure if you're ready for this, Sam. But I think you might be," I hear myself saying as I shift my chair towards the sun.

Sam turns the chair to face me. Looks at me attentively.

I feel a bit nervous. Clench my fists as I say, "I don't think the world we're living in is real."

Sam leans towards me. "You mean this is make-believe?"

Sam believes me. I can feel it. I go on, "I mean I think our thoughts are make-believe. They aren't ours. Well, they are ours to begin with, but then they're taken away from us. Or we just give them away."

Sam gently takes my hands. They're surprisingly cold, like slabs of concrete in the shade, but somehow still warm. "Are you saying you aren't in control of your thoughts?" Their voice is so gentle.

"I'm saying no one is in control of their thoughts."

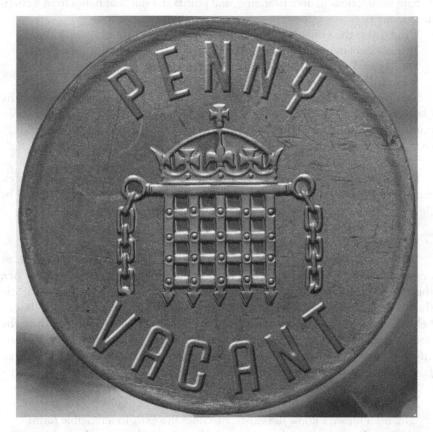

Figure 3.1 "A Penny Vacant"

Artwork produced by the band Penny Vacant, taken during Behind the Noise in 2019. Shared with Measuring Humanity.

Still holding my hands, Sam leans in further, just about whispering in my left ear. "And if you were in control of your thoughts – of everyone's thoughts – what would you do?"

"You mean if I were in charge?"

"If you were in charge."

A flock of geese glides by, their leader headed straight for the sun.

"If I were the Empress of the Thought Empire . . .," I say, waiting for the words to eject from my brain, to land on the tip of my tongue. "If I were the Empress of the Thought Empire . . ." The words arrive. "I would go around telling people they're already free."

"We're already free."

"You're already free."

Sam smiles, nods in understanding, and points at a star that hangs from a chain around my neck.

"And this is the symbol of your Empire, my Empress? Your Gateway?"

Tiny sticks of dynamite detonate in my mind.

"Yes! How do you know about the Gateway?"

"I can feel it. Tell me more about the Thought Empire, then."

Sam gets it. They really get it. I go on, "Well . . . this symbol represents the Gateway between the mortal world and the spiritual realm. Each of the seven points stands for a path of the Higher Self to get you ready for the Otherworld . . . so there's Powers of the Mind and Science, Unconditional Love, Harmony . . ."

"And how do you know which way it faces?"

I'm amazed by Sam's desire for details. "It doesn't matter which way it faces, Sam. It is what you make of it, that's the point. A life philosophy. Inspired by Pine Marten Pat."

"Pine Marten Pat?"

Sam's staring at the star, lured by every syllable.

"Pine Marten Pat. She's a petite Pine Marten. A Pine Martenette. Almost orange. Lies on a small yellow dinghy floating in the ocean. All around her, there's water everywhere. No land in sight. And it's sunny. A bit like today. So she's wearing her black sunglasses, squinting at the sun. Hands casually clasped behind her head as if she doesn't have a care in the world. And the truth is, she doesn't, because she has a theory. A mantra, if you like." I pause for dramatic effect, take a deep breath. "*In search of truth and destiny, she flees The Futile Forest fast. Surrendering to the journey, she finds total freedom at last.*"[55]

Sam's captivated. "So does Pine Marten Pat actually exist?"

A bold but stupid question. "Of course she exists!"

"No, no. I mean, I know she exists. But does she exist in a tangible form?"

"Ah, yes. I see where you're going with this, Sam. We spoke about this in The Community and decided to make her real. Mary moulded a statuette of her out of clay. So now, she exists in real life and lives in our spiritual home in The Futile Forest. That way, we can see her every day and honour her greatness, while we try to make sense of life."

I search Sam's eyes for the usual look that comes when I tell an outsider about my truth. Scorn disguised by interest. Pity covered up by a patronising stare.

But Sam's face isn't giving those thoughts away. There's an openness and acceptance.

I try to think of a word to capture this moment. There is only one.

Magical.

***

INTERLUDE – THE POWER OF IMAGINATION

As I enter my imaginary world through a creative (non)fiction story called "Pork Power," I think about the power of imagination and the extent to which it belongs in public health discourses.

I'm wavering about whether to interrupt this chapter with Pork Power, whether to include this at all, thinking about how exposing and unnerving it feels to experiment with words and data in this way.

I've been reading Phil Crockett Thomas's (2020) work, in particular her collaborative writing of sociological crime fiction to unpack fraud, criminal acts, and criminalisation. Her research troubles taken-for-granted beliefs and explanations of delinquency and offending through creative writing that conveys the complexities and entanglements of the social justice system. It's powerful.

When Thomas quotes novelist Ursula Le Guin, it feels like a prompt. Some food for thought. "The exercise of imagination," she says, "is dangerous to those who profit from the way things are because it has the power to show that the way things are is not permanent, not universal, not necessary" (Thomas 2020).[56]

I decide to go for it.

"PORK POWER"

I love mini pork sausages. They're my absolute favourite. There's a waft of them on the seventh floor, seducing me as I step out of the lift.

"After you."

Ms Marconi holds the silver sliding doors open, gestures in the direction of my temptress. My heeled boots smack against the iciest of tiles, clean enough to eat from. *Thwack, thwack, thwack, thwack.* If this were a secret operation, my cover would have been blown. How can the tiniest of humans make such a racket? I wonder.

I sneak a peek at my chaperon's shoes. Pins for heels, triangles for toes. Yet she's floating. Effortlessly. Carried by a cloud of class, an air of arrival. I wonder if her feet look like mine, lumpy and calloused, with a recurring bout of athlete's foot and an infected right baby toenail that my doctor told me is only going to get worse.

"Did you have a good trip in?"

It's the second time she's tried to make conversation. The first was after I was signed in at the main reception, before I was handed my laminated guest badge announcing that I was not an imposter or a spy.

In between, I'd waited in the echoing lobby. Empty except for one swivelling bucket seat, two bespoke dining chairs with the highest backs I've ever seen, a giant stone pretending to be a coffee table, four glossy magazines (two of them company brochures), and a vase filled with about a dozen lilies.

It all looked and felt familiar. Much like the firm I'd visited the week before.

"My trip was fine, thanks," I say.

The flight itself was uneventful. I hadn't slept the night before, though. Or the night before that. I was in the throes of my most recent episode of insomnia, which had appeared unannounced and uninvited since the onset of this project, much like the virus on the soles of my feet.

We weave our way through marbled corridors lined with cut-glass offices with frosting for walls. Each one looks identical. Clinical. Unused.

"Here we are."

A pristine person in the whitest, tightest pencil skirt is standing outside a glass cube infused with the distinct scent of pan-fried pig. I know I shouldn't judge, but

I'm always slightly suspicious of people who wear white. It's just too impractical a colour for life.

"Hello, welcome. I'm Dr Damira." A shaking of hands. "We took the liberty of ordering lunch. I hope you're hungry."

Starving. I've been on the move since 6:00 a.m., too nervous to eat. I've done this sort of thing a number of times, but today feels different. Significant.

"No, I'm fine, thanks. I grabbed something on the way over."

My stomach growls. I hate lying, but telling the truth isn't an option here. I simply can't touch this food.

"Well, I hope you don't mind if we tuck in, then."

"No, no. Please do. Go ahead."

I don't normally get fed at interviews, particularly when I'm the one doing the interviewing.

A server in a pressed uniform, also white, is waiting by the silver buffet cart she's just rolled in. Shiny metal lids are lifted to reveal a scattering of miniature canapés. Must be a special occasion. Lunchtime on a Tuesday. She looks down shyly as she shuffles out, closing the door behind her. Where's she going? Is there an industrial-sized kitchen somewhere in the building to keep the directors going? A Michelin-starred restaurant in the penthouse?

I hover aimlessly by the foie gras bites and those perfect little pork sausages on sticks, my two hosts towering over me, cherry-picking batons of cucumber and carrot and celery, one at a time, one at a time. I'm conscious of time; I have a late-afternoon flight back home, but no one appears to be in a rush.

"So this is how the other half live," I hear myself say as we take our seats at the glass-and-chrome table. Did those words just come out my mouth, or did I mumble them in my head?

They smile simultaneously.

"Sure." Dr Damira nibbles on a carrot. "You should keep an eye out for jobs. We're advertising quite a lot at the moment. I'm sure someone with your background will be very suitable for this work."

Is this conversation actually happening? I think this is happening, but I am tired. Exhausted even. Maybe I'm hearing things.

Imagine the scandal. Lured from Public Health to Big Tobacco by Little Pigs on Sticks.

I reach for research information sheets and consent forms in my dirty fabric book bag. The kind they give you for free sometimes with a Sunday newspaper. The kind you use as your bag for life when you do your weekly shop. Or when you're meeting tobacco corporate executives, clearly.

I feel dirty and underdressed.

My "smart clothes," a fitted black shirt and knee-length skirt (a different shade of black), have been washed too many times to pass for clean. I, too, have washed, about nine hours ago. In the airport toilet, I splashed cold water on my face and underarms, applied eyeliner with shaking hands to make me feel fierce. Not quite having the desired effect. And I defy any deodorant to shield off the slicks of angst soaking my armpits. This is why you should never wear white.

I watch as Dr Damira, the more mature of the two, dabs a napkin on her tinted lips. Her manicured fingertips, square and crimson, dance at the corner of her mouth for a moment. I'm blinded by the bling on her left ring finger.

My miniature hands, clenched and clammy, are strategically placed under my bum. I don't want them to see cuticles climbing halfway up my nails, the thin layer of filth that refuses to be filed or bitten away.

"I flew in from Madrid this morning," she continues. "I do this a couple of times a week at least. It's part of the job. Busy, always on the move, but I wouldn't have it any other way. I love what I do."

I believe her. Beneath the fine lines and dark rings delicately disguised by layer upon layer of concealer, she looks content. Excited even.

"This is the greatest moment of my career," she says, as if accepting a lifetime achievement award. "I feel like it's all been building to this pinnacle, at last the opportunity to do something incredible. To literally save lives."

The crowds go wild. Ms Marconi springs to her feet for a standing ovation, nodding in unison.

I'm nodding too. Yes, this is an incredible moment in history, I'm sure many in public health would agree. Tobacco companies selling cigarettes that kill on the one hand, and electronic ones that save lives on the other. Tobacco companies holding the curse and the cure. The problem and the solution. And making money from both. It's hard to believe this is real.

Ms Marconi clears her throat. Can she hear my thoughts? She's sitting quietly, hasn't said a word since we've entered the porky incubator. Why is she even here? Is she just meat in the room?

Slightly wearier, she still manages to pull off the straight lines and stitched cuffs. Her charcoal blazer sits on her shoulders exactly where it's meant to. Mine dangles nearer my elbows despite being the smallest size manufacturers dare darn to – a petite 6. A child in adult's clothes playing dress up – that's what I look like as I sit here, waiting to interview two corporate giants. The enormity of the task hits me. My heart plunges to my throat, pulses in my mouth, grips my vocal cords. I'm momentarily mute.

It'll pass. This, too, will pass, I remind myself. Focus on the silent one, the one who looks like she's juggling a demanding corporate job and raising a young family. Imagine her responding to emails from researchers and journalists after midnight between breastfeeding and stolen sleep. All she wants is to have more than four consecutive hours in her bed, much like you, but there's pressure from every angle.

Sales targets, business strategies, corporate social responsibility, nappies, crisis management, risk management, public relations, paying the mortgage, media, social media, lobbying, marriage counselling. Working to maximise shareholder value, to minimise relationship breakdown. Working towards a work-life balance.

"So I thought we'd start with a bit of background. I can tell you a bit more about me and how I came to be in this position," Dr Damira says.

Hold up, I thought I was the one doing the interviewing here? I don't say.

"Sure, go right ahead. I'll start recording."

I'd practiced this fifteen times in the garden across the street from the sky-scraper I'm in. Arrived half an hour early, enough time to get lost and found, to buy a lukewarm take-away coffee from the deli nearby, to pace from bush to park bench, bench to bush.

I start recording. Rummage in my book bag for my bottle of water that was evidently in the pocket of the seat in front on me the plane.

Great. No water, a ninety-minute interview.

There's a large glass of bottled, branded water on the table in front of me. Can I drink the trademarked H_2O? Will I be accused of being on the take? I didn't touch the fancy finger food, but is sipping their water acceptable?

I realise I'm having this conversation about ethics with myself while Dr Damira continues with her life story, which I'm now missing. I'm too busy reliving flash-backs of the time I was asked by a public health academic if hanging out with neoliberals at an e-cigarette event was part of my research.

It was. I was attending to find out what the tobacco industry was saying about e-cigarettes and to meet gatekeepers or potential interviewees for a study we'd received funding for on the condition that we included industry interviews in the study design.

But some people in public health were appalled by the idea of someone like me (usually in the Public Health Goodies camp) speaking to the Baddies. And with good reason. I was suspicious too.

Right now, as I sit slightly nauseated in interview 13, it feels like the most com-plicated thing I've ever done. I remember an exchange with an industry consult-ant who'd invited me to a fancy dinner hosted by a tobacco company.

"Thanks, but no thanks," was my firm reply. "Hospitality doesn't sit comfort-ably with me, and I wouldn't want to do anything to compromise my research."

"I think I do understand," came the response. "Perception really is nine-tenths of reality."

It hadn't stopped the invitations from coming in.

I wonder now, as I sit here in this corporate glass cube, if the perception of me interviewing industry giants on their e-cigarettes business strategies will be that my views are aligned with theirs. When it comes to publishing this data, I won-der, Will we be accused of parroting industry aspirations?

> *Flash forward five years – as it turns out, we would. Even though our critical views on this topic had us firmly placed in the anti-e-cigarette camp. Even though, according to the media, I'd said e-cigarettes encourage children to smoke (I hadn't, but that's what it now says on my research profile). Even though my colleagues and I, who'd expressed scepticism about the products in the early days, had been compared to murderers for wanting smokers to keep smoking real cigarettes.*

I'm back in the room. It still smells of piglet.

"We have a duty, especially on this one . . . where there's so much uncer-tainty in the health community as to whether they'll be good or bad, that we will publish, absolutely publish on this one," Dr D declared. "It's the research and development to make products which are less harmful and which have substantiation that they are less harmful, so I mean, proof, basically, evidence, independently verified and so forth and so on. That's going to be the key."[57]

Dr M worked me through the list of things they're investing in: "Scientists, developing products, doing clinical trials, substantiation of it, and so forth and so on. Research, classic research and development. It is important, especially with the history of the industry, to have very solid science, independently verified."

I assume by "the history of the industry" she's referring to its sordid past, pieced together by thousands of internal tobacco industry documents released through litigation and whistle-blowers revealing the most astonishing systematic corporate deceit of all time. I catch myself reminiscing about the Tobacco Industry Research Committee, a group carefully shaped by a leading public relations firm in the fifties "to serve the industry's collective interests . . . explicitly developed to sustain claims of independence, commitment to science, and pursuit of the 'truth' about tobacco" (Brandt 2012).

My mind drifts to an episode of *Mad Men*. I imagine a vapour-sucking rather than chain-smoking Don Draper in the lead role.

Dr M clears her throat to ensure she has my full and undivided attention. She assures me they're telling the truth, the whole truth, and nothing but the truth. I can check for myself.

"These days, all science documents are publicly available online. It's open to all scrutiny . . . we invite researchers to scrutinise and critique," she continues, tapping her perfect fingertips on the glass table. "We produce millions of pages of high-quality scientific research."

That can't be easy reading, unless there's a mega-University research consortium out there with a lot of time and a lot of money on its hands painstakingly going through each of these millions of pages. One at a time, one at a time. Maybe, in some science-fiction novella, health regulators have the capacity to do these checks (unlike those in the real world)[58] and are verifying these millions of pages, one at a time, one at a time.

"This is where we would like to work with public health, with regulators who have an interest in reduced risk to find out what is the appropriate regulatory path . . . so we are investing a huge amount of time, resource, expertise in the science to enable those conversations and to objectively look at the best route forward."

There's that word again. *Objective*. It's come up in our studies over and over again. I picture myself writing up this research, perhaps in the form of creative (non)fiction, in a completely unbiased way. Unaffected by what I'm experiencing here.

Dr M continues: "I think there is a clear lack of legitimacy and trust that society or regulators have in the tobacco industry as such. I think there are valid reasons for that. You know, we cannot change the past." I wonder if she can read my mind. "We need to look at the future. I don't think people will trust us overnight, but what I would hope is that people can listen to what we say and measure our actions and then draw their own conclusions. Again, we are doing this, you know, as we are a business, we are a very profitable business. We think this makes business sense, but the impact will be, I think, very positive for public health. Like I said, you know, one of the big opportunities in the tobacco industry for a long, long time has been to make products that are less harmful, and I think it's also our . . . moral duty. So if you know that your product is that harmful, try and fix it. I wish more companies would do that, outside the tobacco industry as well. But I think, I can't complain about other companies. I think we need to fix our problems first . . ."

I'm beyond parched. I take a sip of the branded water. It turns into a gulp. I feel like a traitor.

"It's one of those rare occasions, for us, with the Venn diagrams, you know, all the different things can overlap, so there's obviously a business imperative here, to be a sustainable business model going forward. There's a product which is being demanded by adult smokers, and it's fulfilling an aim for public health, which is to find less-harmful ways for people to consume nicotine, because cigarettes are just so uniquely harmful that the status quo is not a particularly attractive proposition," Dr M rounds off.

They flash pearly whites at each other, wait for my next question.

My eyes are burning. My stomach growls. I've been here longer than expected already, but something is still nagging me.

"So my last question is just about targeting. I think you've already covered this before. Your targeting strategies would be . . ."

"Smokers."

"Smokers. Existing smokers only?"

"Yeah."

"Okay. And your business strategy, in relation to that, just to recap, is to switch them."

"Absolutely."

"Okay"

"1.1 billion smokers. It's a big task," Dr D reminds me.

"That is a big task. Well . . . I'm not a business expert, but what I'm wondering is what happens if all of them eventually die of old age."

The room falls silent.

"Look, I think there will continue to be people who start using nicotine products," Dr D finally answers.

I reach to stop the recorder, then one of them says something that scares me. There's no recording of it, no evidence that it even happens, so I can't say if it is real or if I've imagined it. It feels like a threat, but then again so did the whole interview – the whole series of interviews, the whole data collection, analysis, and publishing experience.

All I remember is sprinting from the glass box of a building, shaking, drenched in dread, with a familiar feeling. Much like the one that had settled in after I published on measures to improve transparency of research funding in a leading medical journal (de Andrade 2009). Much like the feeling when my colleagues and I received a legal letter (via our funder, via our University) from a company threatening us for implying something inaccurate and potentially libellous after the publication of a different report. Much like the feeling when I transitioned from journalist to academic investigating the role of power in public health and, when "subjected to personal pressure and implied suggestions of legality," became "inhibited by an all-encompassing fear." A fear that my body remembers. Lodged in my muscle fibres[59] is something I hyperbolically – or realistically? – described as "neurosis . . . turned into full blown paranoia" when contemplating what felt like a real threat of legal action (de Andrade 2014).[60]

That's the thing about corporate power. It's one thing theorising about it (Farnsworth and Holden 2006) or calling it a "psychopath" (Bakan 2005) or calling out those "powerful individuals gliding between the political, corporate and media worlds" with "vested interest[s] in an ideology that furthers corporate interests" (Jones 2015) or throwing stones at them from an ivory tower.

But it's only when you're in its glass building that the crystal catches the sun's rays. And when the beam pierces your skin, when you get burnt, you have a choice. To gallantly step towards Goliath, quivering head held high.

Or to step away, quietly, with your tail between your legs.

Option 2 is the path of least resistance.

Maybe that's one of the reasons systemic issues perpetuate.

***

Notes

1 From the podcast *Poetry Unbound* with Pádraig Ó Tuama, episode "Elizabeth Bishop—Sestina" issued 12 November 2021, by On Being, www.onbeing.org

2 Definition taken from the online *Cambridge English Dictionary*. Accessed 12/11/2021. Available here: ALMANAC | meaning in the Cambridge English Dictionary.

3 Page 112.

4 I use footnotes throughout to give you an insight into the inner workings of my mind as I flip-flop between a creative and relational (creative-relational) analysis and a more conventional approach to analysing data. Sometimes extensive, these comments – or *asides* – are little thought bubbles presented on the page in the form of words (rather than illustrations) as they arrive (there may be an odd picture when words fail me). At times raw and flowing from one thought to the next, these words are my stream of consciousness. A "traditional" public health researcher might view these as "field notes" interspersed with references to theory along the way. This "messiness" or "self-talk" isn't usually presented in published public health texts, but these reflexive notes are integral to my argument. I'm making transparent the ideas, feelings, and beliefs that pop into my mind as I analyse and lead me to "conclusions" that ultimately inform further research, policy, and practice. This internal voice is alive in every researcher. Pretending we can't hear it and cutting it out of public health research can only take us so far.

5 Trying to present nonlinear research – or "ordered complexity" – in a linear way is tricky business. There's a colossal amount of creative ways this may be possible in other media (film, audio, images, performances, or other art forms). But (coherent) written texts require some ordering, so I use footnotes to untangle complex thought processes as they surface, in as simplistic a manner as possible. Flipping from text to footnote, from text to footnote, from text to footnote may be distracting. Or it may

be enriching. Perhaps first read sections in their entirety without footnotes, then with footnotes, and notice how meanings change.

6 Above all, follow your intuition.

7 This is the full moon sometimes referred to as Buddha's birthday. It observes and celebrates birth, enlightenment, and death of the "original" Buddha, Siddhartha Gautama. This isn't a book about Buddhism or religion, though spirituality (defined in many different ways) came up as a theme (that I desperately tried to "code" and "analyse" using traditional public health methods) in just about all the studies presented. I would've preferred to avoid this analysis altogether. Speaking about spirituality or the "soul" in public health, as Hustedde (1998) puts it on page 154 of his article "On the Soul of Community Development," *"raise[s] some eyebrows or cause[s] you to shift a bit in your seat."* I'm sorry if it makes you squirm too. I invite you to stick with the discomfort.

8 I first came across the term *becoming* when I, one of the Applied Social Science researchers, joined the counsellors and psychotherapists in my university department. Our "becoming" (used here in what could be the "right" context – or not) was Counselling, Psychotherapy, and Applied Social Sciences (CPASS). I absolutely felt like an -ASS when words like "becoming" popped up in most conversations along with "I feel" and "fantasy" (in your mind, not as in fantasy the genre, though a fantasy in your mind could be intertwined with fantastical storytelling much like the argument in this book). Anyway, these words "arrived" (another counselling and psychotherapy-ism related to taking your time to "arrive" in the space, the therapy room or Zoom room these days), rather than rushing to speak to fill the awkward silence that usually happens when you first meet and greet someone on the street, and *especially* happens when you first meet and greet someone right in your face on Zoom. Anyway, these words arrived, and I realised I had no idea of their context. A myriad of definitions for *becoming*, long before Michelle Obama claimed it much like the year 2020 claimed the word *lockdown*, will unfold in the chapters that follow. For now, I refer to it as the prospect of transformation in some sort of "thing" that *is*. I'm sure I'll get pelters for this, but maybe later on I'll cite "proper" academic texts to soften the blows.

9 Re-reading this now with my "left brain" firmly in the driving seat – the one that's like a road map, a clear, logical, methodological, and analytical path (or, if you'll indulge my creative "right brain" for a moment, my public health hemisphere) – I sense I'm subconsciously working through theories relating to "affect" and "embodiment." Trying to make sense of them and how they might nourish my work in public health. More on this later.

10 Invisibility – powerlessness – is a relentlessly powerful, recurring theme in this book.

11 An echo chamber (also the working title for a previous iteration of this book, as you'll soon learn) is that place you go to in order to hear yourself being validated. That figurative place where people nod in unison or high-five you when you say something that would cause other people to throw figurative (sometimes real) stones at you. This book, aimed at public health researchers and students, is firmly *not* in an echo chamber. Rocks are ricocheting off me as I type.

12 Liminal space. The "space" between two realities. A concept that's been applied in so many health settings (several cited below) to mean so many things. Graeme Laurie's (Laurie 2017) application of liminality on the limits of law in health research regulation makes me think a comparable paradigm shift in public health research, practice, and policy is possible.

13 I'm Programme Director for an innovative MSc by Research in Health Humanities and Arts that explores health and well-being through the lens of arts and humanities practice and knowledge. Paul Crawford (Crawford et al. 2015) coined *health humanities* as a discipline distinct to medical humanities. It includes "non-medical" people related to health, such as allied health workers, nurses, patients, and carers.

14 The hyphen – appearing in the oddest of places. In the last couple of years, I learnt that some academics have made entire careers out this little line between words. Jonathan Wyatt brought this to my attention when he created Creative-Relational Inquiry. I then read Michelle Fine's work (Fine 1994). Flash forward a few years and I would find myself writing with Jonathan and Rosie Stenhouse, citing the word *hyphen* thirty-one times in a paper pushing further "at the engagement between the creative, the relational, and the hyphen that binds them, and how it might provide a nuanced effort to problematize, and provide alternatives for, taken-for-granted assumptions concerning research and research practices" (de Andrade, Stenhouse, and Wyatt 2020) (page 1).

15 Article 5.3 of the World Health Organization Framework Convention on Tobacco Control says "there is a fundamental and irreconcilable conflict between the tobacco industry's interests and public health policy interests. . . . The broad array of strategies and tactics used by the tobacco industry to interfere with the setting and implementing of tobacco control measures . . . is documented by a vast body of evidence. The measures recommended in these guidelines aim at protecting against interference not only by the tobacco industry but also, as appropriate, by organizations and individuals that work to further the interests of the tobacco industry." A conditional offer response from our funder noted that "the proposal would benefit from speaking to people responsible for marketing the products themselves, or creating their marketing strategies."

16 REF: the system for assessing the quality of research in UK higher education institutions. I can't even begin to get into the politics of this one. Will this book even count for the next REF? I bloody well hope so! Blood, sweat, and actual tears *should* count as proper research.

17 Six things I've learnt about studying the system:

1. You can't throw yourself at the system. Like a spitting snake, it'll swallow you whole but spit you out in pieces.
2. If you dig deep and discover the "truth" of the system, you aren't blinded by the light you have seen. There's a darkness that lives there.
3. If you sit in that darkness first for a day, then a week, for a year, many years . . . you become that darkness. You become its shadow.
4. A shadow of your former self, you resist at first then slowly start to see a reflection of yourself in the system. Its attributes feel strangely familiar.
5. Just when you think you've figured the system out, it changes. Like an amorphous beast, it shape-shifts.

18 These handheld devices heat a liquid to produce a vapour that users (or vapours) inhale. As these products tend to contain nicotine (some don't) but not tobacco (some do), they are generally considered to be safer than smoking and are being promoted (by some) as safe and effective tobacco-harm-reduction devices. The last time I researched this, there was still much debate and uncertainty. See for example (The Lancet 2019; Newton 2019).

19 I realise I'm now writing a book within a book within a book. It's all connected.

20 Page 473.

21 Spinoza, Deleuze, Massumi, Sedgwick, and Ahmed are some key scholars of affect. Distinct from emotions, which, according to page 177 in "Affect: An Introduction" by Daniel White, are "feelings that fix into place through a variety of discursive practices," affect is concerned with "nonconscious entities" (quoting (Massumi 2002)) and "renders capture impossible." Blackman notes, "Affect is disclosed in atmospheres, fleeting fragments and traces, gut feelings and embodied reactions and in felt intensities and sensations. Affect is performed in practices and modulated within techniques, which exceed discrete bounded individuated human bodies" (Blackman 2007; White 2017).

22 Behind the Noise (BTN) is a COSLA Award–winning and SQA-accredited music and skills programme (http://behindthenoise.co.uk/education/). I collaborated with BTN in *Measuring Humanity through Music in Schools* to apply the Asset-Based Indicator Framework (ABIF) in secondary schools, including in areas of multiple deprivation. We engaged more than 100 participants (sixteen- to eighteen-year-olds) in fourteen mainstream schools and three assisted-learning schools. BTN aims to inspire, encourage, and support young people who have an interest in music and the various career and further learning opportunities that exist within the creative sector. It's delivered by industry professionals via a series of workshops, rehearsal days, recording sessions, industry panels and culminates in a run of live events where pupils not only perform but also assist in promoting and delivering all aspects of the shows. Prior to engaging with Measuring Humanity, BTN had been collecting evidence – mostly in the form of surveys and case studies – for four years. They also had data on ex-students putting on shows over a three-month sample period and hundreds of recorded tracks on SoundCloud with around a third being original. Impact for BTN had been focused on creativity, confidence, and employability. By working with Measuring Humanity, the aim was to evidence (i) how the project may also be improving health and well-being for school children from these disadvantaged neighbourhoods and (ii) how it can help shape related local and national policies. The idea was for ABIF workshops to be applied from baseline, tracking changes in health indicators from the start of the project up until its completion. As with other ABIF applications, impact was to be evidenced through the framework itself and ensuing interviews, questionnaires, surveys, and films alongside innovative approaches to evidence – the music outputs themselves. But as was the case with *Measuring Humanity in Green Spaces*, we were left wanting after analysing data using traditional public health approaches. The most compelling data we collected was the music itself – the lyrics and notes – and, perhaps more importantly, the process of "getting behind" the lyrics and notes to connect with aspiring young musicians as they created performing art. Getting Behind the Noise to feel our way through our findings.

23 From now on, imagine that Behind the Noise is the soundtrack to this book. Imagine you're part of an immersive reading experience that allows you to both read the words on this page and also hear the music being referred to in the text. In fact, no need to imagine it. If you're reading the electronic version of this book, why not play the song in the background so you can get a sense of what's going on for Sara and Sam? So you can get a sense of the music created by musicians in Behind the Noise. Here's the first tune to our soundtrack: Listen to "Complications" by källa (Gryffe High School) by Behind the Noise in Sessions 2018/19 playlist online for free on SoundCloud. https://soundcloud.com/behindthenoise/complications-by-kalla-gryffe-high-school

24 These are the actual lyrics in "Complications" by källa. Later on in the book, you'll see how we tried to analyse these words to make sense of the young musicians' experiences of health and well-being. To make sense of their inner world. To make sense of their reality. So we could use it to evidence positive changes in health. You'll also see how futile the exercise was.

25 Still citing the lyrics here.

26 Citing the prolific psychiatrist and psychoanalyst Carl Jung, the Religious Studies scholar Leon Schlamm states, "Numinous experiences, identified by Jung with experiences of the unconscious . . . possess a 'deeply stirring emotional effect' . . . 'thrilling power' . . . *mana* (psychic power) equated with holiness, healing or destructive qualities . . . and are therefore unusually persuasive from the psychological point of view. . . . They are independent of conscious volition, transporting 'the subject into the state of rapture, which is a state of will-less surrender.' . . . For this reason, they are 'difficult to handle intellectually, since our affectivity is involved . . . absolute objectivity is more rarely achieved here than anywhere else'" (Schlamm 2008) (page 2).

27 Vignettes are brief stories about hypothetical characters in imagined circumstances. Interviewees are asked to respond to these conditions to gain more insight into the topic under investigation (Finch 1987).

28 Page x.

29 Page xii.

30 Page 26.

31 Page 243.

32 Page 38.

33 Page 90.

34 Are the Sphere-Blue Drive (mind) and Emotion-Defibrillator © (body) implants real or unreal? Ethical or immoral? Acceptable or deplorable?

35 Page 6.

36 This is the focus of the Centre for Creative-Relational Inquiry as defined on our website (The University of Edinburgh 2021). Accessed 15/11/2021. Available here: Centre for Creative-Relational Inquiry | The University of Edinburgh.

37 Page 11.

38 The Pragmatic Theory of Truth (Stanford Encyclopedia of Philosophy 2019). Accessed 17/11/2021. Available here: The Pragmatic Theory of Truth (Stanford Encyclopedia of Philosophy).

39 Page 105.

40 Pages 6, 11.

41 Page 10.

42 Page 961

43 Page 962.

44 Ibid.

45 Page 963.

46 BBC Bitesize: Animal Farm Plot Summary (2022). Accessed 14/11/2021. Available here: Animal Farm - Plot summary - Plot summary - GCSE English Literature Revision - BBC Bitesize.

47 The Pragmatic Theory of Truth (Stanford Encyclopedia of Philosophy 2019). Accessed 17/11/2021. Available here: The Pragmatic Theory of Truth (Stanford Encyclopedia of Philosophy).

48 I'm thinking about Barnfield's (2016) "fundamental notion of affect," that is, "the capacity to affect and to be affected. A body being able to affect and be affected by another body. It necessitates an encounter, a state of already being immersed in the world." (Page 3.)

49 The philosopher Alan Watts says we need to "become more intensely aware of the living vibrations of the real world." Rather than *thinking* about what a text is telling us through *description*, try to get in touch with the *sensations* being created within a narrative and how they bring about different meanings (Watts 2010). (Page xii.)

50 This resonates with *Vibrant Matter* by Professor of Humanities Jane Bennett, who invites us to be with "a cultivated, patient, sensory attentiveness to nonhuman forces operating outside and inside the human body" (Bennett 2010). (Page xiv.)

51 I'm influenced by performative approaches to representation "that moves outside analytic/logical and emotional embodied distinctions to 'make possible' other identities, discourses, and ways of living and relating." In *Creative Selves/Creative Cultures* (Holman Jones 2018), Stacey Holman Jones and Marc Pruyn, citing Della Pollock, invite us to embrace "the partial, incomplete, unspeakable, and immaterial in selves and cultures alongside our efforts to write and represent our-selves and our communities in relation." (Page 11.)

52 Here I'm stirred by page 218 of *Creative Selves/Creative Cultures* (Holman Jones 2018), where performer and researcher Phoebe Green describes her autoethnographic writing – *Creating Memories: A Cartography of Musical Learning* – as "a catalyst for

memory and remembering; auditory, kinetic, sensorial and emotional, revealing insights into what is otherwise an invisible process."

53 Words from the original song by Penny Vacant created for Behind the Noise. Feel free to immerse yourself in the audio recording here: Listen to "Not Quite What You Expected" by Penny Vacant (Glennifer High School) by Behind the Noise in Sessions 2018/19 playlist online for free on SoundCloud. https://soundcloud.com/behindthenoise/not-quite-what-you-expected-by

54 This is the original artwork created by the band Penny Vacant in Behind the Noise.

55 I'm inspired by the artist Edward Monkton and his creation, *Zen Dog*, that I found on a hallmark card. Accessed 20/11/2021. Available here: Edward Monkton - Gallery.

56 Page 220.

57 Much of the dialogue in this scene is made up of direct quotes from "real" interviews with tobacco executives.

58 A 2007 report on the US health regulator, the Food and Drug Administration's "oversight of clinical trials" found that it investigated only 1 percent of clinical trial sites (Levinson 2007). A House of Commons Inquiry into the Influence of the Pharmaceutical Industry raised similar concerns regarding failures of the UK health regulator (House of Commons Health Committee 2005).

59 Here, I draw this imagery from page 39 of the by Michel Foucault, who vividly illustrates that power's "reality" is local, capillary, and reaches "into the very grain of individuals, touches their bodies and inserts itself into their actions and attitudes, their discourses, learning processes and everyday lives" (Foucault 1890).

60 Page 18.

References

Bakan, Joel. 2005. *The Corporation: The Pathological Pursuit of Profit and Power*. Toronto: The Penguin Group.

Barad, Karen. 2007. "Meeting the Universe Halfway: Quantum Physics and the Entanglement of Matter and Meaning." *Meeting the Universe Halfway*: 140–223. https://doi.org/10.1215/9780822388128.

———. 2010. "Quantum Entanglements and Hauntological Relations of Inheritance: Dis/Continuities, Spacetime Enfoldings, and Justice to Come." *Derrida Today* 3 (2): 240–68. https://doi.org/10.3366/E1754850010000813.

Barnfield, Andrew. 2016. "Affect and Public Health – Choreographing Atmospheres of Movement and Participation." *Emotion, Space and Society* 20 (August): 1–9. https://doi.org/10.1016/J.EMOSPA.2016.04.003.

Bennett, Jane. 2010. *Vibrant Matter: A Political Ecology of Things*. Durham and London: Duke University Press.

Berwick, D. M. 2005. "Broadening the View of Evidence-Based Medicine." *Quality & Safety in Health Care* 14 (5): 315. https://doi.org/10.1136/QSHC.2005.015669.

Bishop, Elizabeth. 1956. "Sestina." *The New Yorker*. 1956. www.newyorker.com/magazine/1956/09/15/sestina.

Blackman, Lisa. 2007. "Researching Affect and Embodied Hauntologies: Exploring an Analytics of Experimentation." *Affective Methodologies: Developing Cultural Research Strategies for the Study of Affect* (February): 25–44. https://doi.org/10.1057/9781137483195_2.

Brandt, Allan M. 2012. "Inventing Conflicts of Interest: A History of Tobacco Industry Tactics." *American Journal of Public Health* 102 (1): 63. https://doi.org/10.2105/AJPH.2011.300292.

Bruner, Jerome. 1991. *The Narrative Construction of Reality*. Critical Inquiry. 1st ed. Vol. 18. University of Chicago Press. www.jstor.org/stable/1343711.

Caine, Vera, M. Shaun Murphy, Andrew Estefan, D. Jean Clandinin, Pamela Steeves, and Janice Huber. 2016. "Exploring the Purposes of Fictionalization in Narrative Inquiry." 23 (3): 215–21. https://doi.org/10.1177/1077800416643997.

Crawford, Paul, Brian Brown, Charley Baker, Victoria Tischler, and Brian Abrams. 2015. "Health Humanities." *Health Humanities*: 1–19. https://doi.org/10.1057/9781137282613_1.

de Andrade, Marisa de. 2009. "In Clear Sight." Edited by G. Balint, B. Antala, C. Carty, J-M. A. Mabieme, I. B. Amar, and A. Kaplanova. *British Medical Journal* 339 (7720): 339. https://doi.org/10.2/JQUERY.MIN.JS.

———. 2014. "Public Relations and Aca-Media: Autoethnography, Ethics and Engagement in the Pharmaceutical Industry." 3 (1): 113–36. https://doi.org/10.1177/2046147X13519813.

de Andrade, Marisa de, Kathryn Angus, Gerard Hastings, and Nikolina Angelova. 2020. "Hostage to Fortune: An Empirical Study of the Tobacco Industry's Business Strategies since the Advent of e-Cigarettes." *Critical Public Health* 30 (3): 280–93. https://doi.org/10.1080/09581596.2018.1552778/SUPPL_FILE/CCPH_A_1552778_SM6000.PDF

de Andrade, Marisa, and Gerald Hastings. 2013. "Tobacco Harm Reduction and E-Cigarettes: Setting a Unified Research Agenda." *Tobacco Control*. 2013. https://blogs.bmj.com/tc/2013/05/29/tobacco-harm-reduction-and-e-cigarettes-setting-a-unified-research-agenda/.

de Andrade, Marisa de, Gerard Hastings, and Kathryn Angus. 2013. "Promotion of Electronic Cigarettes: Tobacco Marketing Reinvented?" *BMJ* 347 (December): f7473. https://doi.org/10.1136/BMJ.F7473.

de Andrade, Marisa De, Rosie Stenhouse, and Jonathan Wyatt. 2020. "Some Openings, Possibilities, and Constraints of Creative-Relational InquiryIntroduction to the Special Issue." *Departures in Critical Qualitative Research* 9 (2): 1–15. https://doi.org/10.1525/DCQR.2020.9.2.1.

Denzin, Norman, and Yvonna Lincoln. 2005. *The Sage Handbook of Qualitative Research*. 3rd ed. Sage Publications Ltd. https://psycnet.apa.org/record/2005-07735-000.

Ellis, Carolyn, and Arthur P. Bochner. 1996. *Composing Ethnography: Alternative Forms of Qualitative Writing*. 1st ed. Walnut Creek, CA: AltaMira Press.

Farnsworth, Kevin, and Chris Holden. 2006. "The Business-Social Policy Nexus: Corporate Power and Corporate Inputs into Social Policy." *Journal of Social Policy* 35 (3): 473–94. https://doi.org/10.1017/S0047279406009883.

Finch, Janet. 1987. "The Vignette Technique in Survey Research." (July). https://doi.org/10.1177/0038038587021001008.

Fine, Michelle. 1994. "Working the Hyphens: Reinventing Self and Other in Qualitative Research." *Handbook of Qualitative Research*: 70–82. https://psycnet.apa.org/record/1994-98625-003.

Foucault, Michel. 1890. *Power/Knowledge: Selected Interviews and Other Writings*. New York: Pantheon Books.

Frye, Marilyn. 1983. *The Politics of Reality: Essays in Feminist Theory*. Trumansburg, N.Y. CA: Crossing Press.

Gale, Ken, and Jonathan Wyatt. 2018. "Autoethnography and Activism." *Edinburgh Research Explorer* 3. https://doi.org/10.1177/1077800418800754.

Gordon, Avery, and Janice Radway. 2008. *Ghostly Matters: Haunting and the Sociological Imagination*. University of Minnesota Press. https://muse.jhu.edu/book/27669.

Harré, Niki, Barbara Grant, Locke Kirsten, and Sean Strum. 2017. "The University as an Infinite Game: Revitalising Activism in the Academy." *Australian Universities Review* 59 (2): 5–13.

Hoffman, Alice. 2014. *The Museum of Extraordinary Things*. New York: Scribner.

Holman Jones, Stacy. 2018. "Creative Selves/Creative Cultures: Critical Autoethnography, Performance, and Pedagogy." *Creative Selves/Creative Cultures*: 3–20. https://doi.org/10.1007/978-3-319-47527-1_1.

House of Commons Health Committee. 2005. *The Influence of the Pharmaceutical Industry*. London. www.parliament.uk.

Hustedde, Ronald J. 1998. "On the Soul of Community Development." *Journal of the Community Development Society* 29 (2): 153–65.

Jones, Owen. 2015. *The Establishment: And How They Get Away with It*. London: Allen Lane.

The Lancet. 2019. "E-Cigarettes: Time to Realign Our Approach?" *Lancet (London, England)* 394 (10206): 1297. https://doi.org/10.1016/S0140-6736(19)32277-9.

Laurie, Graeme. 2017. "Liminality and the Limits of Law in Health Research Regulation: What Are We Missing in the Spaces in-Between?" *Medical Law Review* 25 (1): 47–72. https://doi.org/10.1093/MEDLAW/FWW029.

Levinson, Daniel R. 2007. "The Food and Drug Administration's Oversight of Clinical Trials." *Department of Health and Human Services: Office of Inspector General*. http://oig.hhs.gov.

Lucherini, Mark. 2018. "Caught in the Middle: Early Career Researchers, Public Health and the Emotional Production of Research." 30 (3): 367–72. https://doi.org/10.1080/09581596.2018.1550252.

Massumi, Brian. 2002. *Parables for the Virtual: Movement, Affect, Sensation*. Durham, NC: Duke University Press.

Mehl-Madrona, Lewis. 2010. *Healing the Mind Through the Power of Story: The Promise of Narrative Psychiatry*. www.amazon.co.uk/Healing-Mind-Through-Power-Story/dp/159143095X.

Mitchell, Susan. 2010. *Spiritual Aspects of Psychosis and Recovery*. Edinburgh: Royal College of Psychiatrists.

Newton, John N. 2019. "Time for The Lancet to Realign with the Evidence on E-Cigarettes?" *Lancet (London, England)* 394 (10211): 1804–5. https://doi.org/10.1016/S0140-6736(19)32486-9.

Orwell, George. 1945. *Animal Farm*. London: Secker and Warburg.

Owton, Helen. 2017. "Doing Poetic Inquiry." *Doing Poetic Inquiry*. https://doi.org/10.1007/978-3-319-64577-3.

Poetry Unbound. 2020. "On Being." https://onbeing.org/programs/welcome-to-poetry-unbound/#:~:text=Poetry Unbound features an immersive exploration of a,on season 2 for release in Fall 2020.

Raimondi, Gustavo Antonio, Claudio Moreira, and Nelson Filice de Barros. 2020. "This Text Is (Not) a Scientific Paper." *Qualitative Inquiry* 26 (7): 931–40. https://doi.org/10.1177/1077800419868510.

Richardson, Laurel. 1990. *Writing Strategies: Reaching Diverse Audiences*. Newbury Park, CA: Sage Publications.

Rodríguez-Dorans, Edgar, Fiona Murray, Marisa de Andrade, Jonathan Wyatt, and Rosie Stenhouse. 2021. "Qualitative Inquiry, Activism, the Academy, and the Infinite Game." *International Review of Qualitative Research* 14 (1). https://doi.org/10.1177/1940844721991079.

Rosiek, J. L., J. Snyder, and S. L. Pratt. 2020. "The New Materialisms and Indigenous Theories of Non-Human Agency: Making the Case for Respectful Anti-Colonial Engagement." *Qualitative Inquiry* 26 (3–4): 331–46. doi:10.1177/1077800419830135

Schlamm, Leon. 2008. "C. G. Jung and Numinous Experience: Between the Known and the Unknown." 9 (4): 403–14. https://doi.org/10.1080/13642530701725981.

Speedy, Jane. 2015. *Staring at the Park: A Poetic Autoethnographic Inquiry*. New York: Routledge.

Stanford Encyclopedia of Philosophy. 2019. *The Pragmatic Theory of Truth*. Stanford, CA: Stanford Encyclopedia of Philosophy.

Stenhouse, Rosemary Clare. 2013. *Unfulfilled Expectations: A Narrative Study of Individuals' Experiences of Being a Patient on an Acute Psychiatric Inpatient Ward in Scotland*. Saarbrucken, Germany: Lambert Academic Publishing. https://era.ed.ac.uk/handle/1842/4071.

———. 2014. "Hearing Voices: Re/Presenting the Findings of Narrative Research into Patient Experience as Poems." *Journal of Psychiatric and Mental Health Nursing* 21 (5): 423–37. https://doi.org/10.1111/JPM.12094.

Thomas, Phil. 2020. "Writing Sociological Crime Fiction: You Will Have You Day in Court." *Art/Research International* 6 (1). https://journals.library.ualberta.ca/ari/index.php/ari/article/view/29549/22024.

The University of Edinburgh. 2021. "Centre for Creative-Relational Inquiry." *School of Health in Social Science*. 2021. www.ed.ac.uk/health/research/centres/ccri.

Vance, Erik. 2016. *Suggestible You: The Curious Science of Your Brain's Ability to Deceive, Transform, and Heal*. Washington, D.C.: National Geographic Partners.

Watts, Alan. 2010. *Does It Matter? Essays on Man's Relation to Materiality*. Novato, CA: New World Library.

White, Daniel. 2017. "Affect: An Introduction." *Cultural Anthropology* 32 (2): 175–80. https://doi.org/10.14506/CA32.2.01.

Wyatt, Jonathan. 2007. "Research, Narrative and Fiction: Conference Story." *The Qualitative Report* 12 (2): 318–31. www.nova.edu/ssss/QR/QR12-2/wyatt.pdf.

———. 2018. *Therapy, Stand-Up, and the Gesture of Writing*. Therapy, Stand-Up, and the Gesture of Writing. Routledge. https://doi.org/10.4324/9781315178790.

Yue, E., L. Llerena, L. Prendergast, and V. Ho. 2021. "Psychosis: Narrative Psychiatry as an Assets-Based Model." In *Humanities and Arts-Informed Methods in the Social Sciences Formative Assessment Presentation*. Edinburgh: School of Health in Social Sciences.

4   Knowledge is power

We rejoin In-Credible, Sara, and sixty-four Community Members sitting around a flickering fire in the majestic Futile Forest on the 212th floor of the infamous Beguile Building, shaped like a ginormous bulbous pear.

The sensor-synchronised 4DX screens turn black. Four-dimensional figures of Sam and Sara fade. They're replaced with an image of a square – a different one – presenting a smorgasbord of visual treats. Boom-boxing street dancers dressed as firefighters, men made of wire bikes made of balloons. A burger joint is hidden behind a group of pygmies dressed as pugs. Or maybe they're just very large pugs.

A track by Half Life Human from Behind the Noise[1] starts blasting from hidden stereos:

> "I know it's too late . . .
>   for all of this to change.
>   Maybe you're the one who's far away.
> Every time I think I'm safe . . .*
>   it comes right back into my face.
> It stays the same.
> Will it ever end?
>   Tell me what you're doing here.
>   You were gone.
> Why did you disappear?"[2]

"What's happening?" I ask Sara as lights come on and The Community starts moving about.

"We're taking a break," she says as she stretches her legs.

"Taking a break? What do you mean? You can't stop like that. I was just getting into this."

"In-Credible, this isn't a film. This is my life. And a methodology book." She points towards the elevator that brought us up here. "If you need the toilet, it's that way."

---

* "As a process of the traumatic imagination, magical realist writing keeps alive the illusion and the mystery inherent in phenomenal knowledge, particularly when the object of that knowledge is death or pain . . ." (Arva 2008).

DOI: 10.4324/9781003196488-4

I head in that direction, then find myself drying my hands in a noisy device that sucks every last drop of moisture from my pores.

I hear a flush, then running water from the tap behind me.

"Excuse me, do you have any hand cream?" I ask the long thin person washing their hands.

They ignore me. Not even a look my way before they head straight out the door, wiping their hands on their trousers.

Another flush, more running water from the tap behind me.

"Excuse me, do you have any hand cream?" I ask the person with black-rimmed glasses washing their hands.

They ignore me. Not even a look my way before they head straight out the door, wiping their hands on their trousers.

What, am I invisible now?

I head out to find Sara seated in front of the bonfire that's blazed up again.

"Some people are being really rude to me," I tell her. "Why are they ignoring me? Do they know who I am and why I'm here?"

"Who's being rude to you?"

I point to the pair.

"They can't hear you," Sara says.

"What do you mean they can't hear me?"

"I mean they can't hear you. They're Deaf."

"They're deaf?"

"They're Deaf, not deaf."

"That's what I said."

"No. You said *deaf* with a small *d*. It's *Deaf* with a capital *D*."

"What's the difference?"

"What do you mean what's the difference?"

"I mean what's the difference. *Deaf* with a capital *D* and *deaf* with a small *d*?"

"Really? You work in health and you don't know the difference?"

"Really. I work in health and I don't know the difference."

"Wow, okay. *Deaf* with a capital *D* is people who've been Deaf all their lives or since before they started to speak. So sign language is their first language."

I look around the blaze, where the sixty-four other Community Members have gathered, some with their eyes closed, others talking animatedly in a language I can't understand, others signing. Incredible. I hadn't noticed.

"So how many Deaf people are there here?"

"Fifteen. And four interpreters. You hadn't noticed?"

I shake my head sheepishly. "And the others are speaking in tongues?" I try to joke.

"Wow. You need to meet Mark Rodger," Sara says and points to someone who's lying on his back. "He's a Deaf comedian. Famous. He might be able to help you out with your one-liners."

I look away, my cheeks stinging.

"Marta over there is speaking Polish to Anna and Lena. Ali's speaking to Arham and Aisha in Urdu. Elena and Dana are speaking to each other in

Romanian. And Magda and Varga are speaking Slovak. You'll have noticed the interpreters . . . ?"

I look away again. How've I missed all this? The details. The granularity. The "thick description."[3]

"So what happens now?" I ask Sara, thinking I could do with a halloumi and hummus wrap. "Aren't you getting hungry?"

"Don't talk about food here. Most of us spend our time at food banks."

I can't look her in the eyes after this.

"What happens now is this . . . take one and pass on."

She hands me a pile of papers. I take one and pass on until we all have a single sheet. I start reading:

4.1 Knowledge is power

Distinctly different groups of people are put in the same [Box] under the newly mandated Homogeneous Humans Health Act, hailed as the most progressive policy of its time. People who (i) look (more or less) the same, (ii) sound as if they may come from the same place (more or less), AND (iii) are *not* the same as natives coexist in the same box – Black Asian Minority Ethnic, or BAME.

When the figures are added up, there is an overwhelming amount of BAMEs (more than eight million). A statutory decision is therefore taken to divide them equally so each [Box] is made up of 100 people dictated by geographical boundaries. The thinking is that by categorising BAMEs in this way, The State can make comparisons (such as rates and averages of characteristics) of public health data to (i) understand more about the causes of diseases and conditions and (ii) detect and tackle health research, policy, and practice inequities evidence in varying outcomes.

In "*Knowledge is power*," we have a bird's-eye view of life in one of these [Boxes] in a city called Hollow. Here, four distinct groups bounce off each other, their cultural characteristics jarring at times. We join them in a community hall one rainy Friday as they try to make sense of their collective identities while firmly holding on to their uniqueness. They are politely appeasing a patronising public health researcher who promised them music, theatre, food, and "fun" and arrives with an entourage of policymakers, health practitioners, and charity workers (who were also promised music, theatre, food, and "fun" – oh, and learning).

The whole set-up is more than a little cringeworthy, but no one notices as they're too busy acting *as if* they're being welcomed into the warmth of a make-believe world where health care is equal for all. As they enact Theatre of the Oppressed (where the audience are spect-actors) for a show called *Come On In!*, you're left confused as to whether life is imitating art, art is imitating life, or everyone's just putting on an act. The end point is a Co-produced Health Service called The Void (fact), which never materialises in the real world (also a fact). Spirituality turns out to be a health outcome that can't be seen, touched, or measured (another fact).

"What's this?" I ask. "It's a bit random."

"It's a peer-reviewed paper we're working on together about a study some of us took part in," Sara replies.

"You're writing a journal paper about your experiences of taking part in an academic study? Are you even allowed to do that? Do you even know how to do that? I mean, who's the PI? Who owns the data from that study? Are any of you even academics?"

I look around at the huddled and bundled bodies warming themselves on an open flame in the fantasy Futile Forest at the top of the Beguile Buildings.

You couldn't make this up.

"We're the 'subjects.' We're scripting this," Sara replies.

***

INTERLUDE – MAKING SENSE OF (NON)METHODOLOGY

When I read Ken Gale's opening lines to his book *Madness as Methodology: Bringing Concepts to Life in Contemporary Theorising and Inquiry*, the dancer in me did a triple pirouette on the inside.

It just made sense to me.

Ken reflects on the process of writing his book, "starting in the middle," and "starting with sense." Conceiving of the text as "onto-episto-methodological," he suggests that "sense" takes him "into the world," "leads" him "to it and is its instrument of creation." "In sensing," Ken posits, "space becomes place, where 'becomes' is always processual, never an end point" (Gale 2018).[4]

Could this post-human theorising as practice help me feel my way through my public health data rather than trying to squeeze into a cognitive reductionist framework?

Ken cites Deleuze and Guattari from the onset – "Madness need not be all breakdown. It may also be breakthrough" (Deleuze and Guattari 2000)[5] – and goes on to conceptualise "madness, not as a condition of an individual or particular being, but rather as a process that does things differently in terms of creativity and world making."

Great. I'm on board. Just tell me how. Tell me how to use and "do" this methodology. Give me the procedural steps that I can give to the readers of this book so they can give it to journal reviewers so they can get four-star papers for REF. Please.

I read. I scan. I read. I land on a "provocative starting point" – Ken is essentially proposing "a non-methodology" (Gale 2018).[6]

Tricky. I can't see public health being on board with this, but I read on.

With reference to Whitehead's (1929) "organic realism," this non-methodological approach rejects "Cartesian Dualisms of mind/body, rationalism/empiricism, subjectivity/objectivity" and engages "with the idea that perception is not simply a representation of the external world but rather it is part of the world." It's a "part-to-whole relationality" that's part of a process (Gale 2018).[7]

I think of how engagement with science in my research – and engagement with various individuals and institutions that are generating that science – has been posited as perception being nine-tenths of reality. The way you think about it, interpret it, or understand it – and the way that science is communicated in peer-reviewed publications that go on to influence policy and practice, the media, and other formal or informal communication channels – has a meaningful impact on others' perception. And construction of reality.

Thinking with Ken, I'm seeing perception *as a part of reality* rather than a representation of it.

This changes everything.

A move away from methodology towards *"methodogenisis*, in which research doings are always becoming and in which conceptualisation and inventive research process is given precedence over the fixities of methodological representation and signification" (Gale 2018).[8]

Research doings.

I feel my research "participants" come alive with these two words put together. I feel them embodying the "futility of trying to capture any movement or moment" with the knowledge that such a methodological approach is shallow, political, and based on preconceived depictions of people and their identities (Gale 2018).[9]

I can hear my "participants" smashing through the categories that were created for them. BAME. Roma. Travellers. Gypsies. Ethnic. Other.

I can see them tearing down the binary walls of categorisation – "sane/insane, rational/irrational, neurotic/psychotic and so on" (Gale 2018).[10]

I can read their (imagined) peer-reviewed paper of a study they took part in and have taken ownership of.

I can imagine them trying to make sense of the ways in which academics are meant to design and analyse studies with the "right" kind of methodology to make it "useful" for public health research, policy, and practice.

***

ORIGINAL ARTICLE ROUTLEDGE

KNOWLEDGE IS POWER:[11] MAKING SENSE OF A
METHODOLOGICAL MESS IN "BAME" HEALTH POLICY
AND PRACTICE

Received: now
Revised: now
Accepted: now
Veritas Journal of Truth, Storytelling, and Science
Authors: Anna, Lena, Marta, Ali, Arham, Aisha, Elena, Dana, Magda, Varga*

*These aren't our real names. They're pseudonyms to protect our identity because we're "vulnerable." This means, as co-authors and "research participants," we can't be known by our real names even though we're writing this. Our names are in no particular order. We picked them out of a hat.

4.1.1 Analysis and ethics

We pick writing as a form of inquiry, a narrative health care of an eth-nodrama (Theatre of the Oppressed) sprinkled with inter-texuality and standpoint theory as a method(s) and analysis framework(s) grounded in post-modernism that leans on post-structuralism. As we were involved in the ethnodrama (as participants and observers) and our research journey began with an ethnography, we cannot separate ourselves from seeing things from "a native point of view" (we are the natives). We therefore have to write ourselves into this work so also need to use (collaborative) autoethnography as a methodology.

We are all distinctly different groups of people – collectively known as BAMES – and have been put in the same [Box] under the newly mandated Homogeneous Humans Health Act because we look and/or sound the same/similar and are/could be from the same place (or thereabout).

We call our methodological approach Reality of the Absurd.[12]

We know we're meant to somehow connect this bricolage, but so far, we accept that this is more than messy. It's a mess.

4.1.2 A methodological mess

This will never do. We'll be slaughtered in peer review.

We need to pick ONE methodology for this to count as an acceptable form of research. Even then, depending on the type of methodology we pick, our knowledge generation may still not count as meaningful research.

We turn to literature again for validation, and for direction, and find this:

> Some speak greedily and urgently about method; method is all they wish to see in their work. It never seems rigorous or formal enough to them. Method becomes Law . . .
>
> (Barthes 1971)

And this:

> Method inevitably disappoints, posing as a pure metalanguage, it partakes of the vanity of all metalanguages. Thus, a work that unceasingly declares its will-to-methodology always becomes sterile in the end. Everything takes place inside the method, nothing is left to the writing. The researcher repeats that his text will be methodological, but this text never arrives. There is nothing more sure to kill research and sweep it off into the left-overs of abandoned works, nothing more sure than method.[13]

We feel lighter and somewhat enlightened but still don't know where to start. How to create structure and order from research findings that are embedded within findings from multiple sources, voices, places, contexts, languages, and histories? Can any methodological framework do this type of inquiry justice?

We start by re-reading direct quotes from the interviews we gave to an excitable researcher. Then we re-read notes from our ethnographic observations. Then we watch nine video clips with highlights from the Theatre of the Oppressed knowledge-exchange event we took part in.

We decide to use each of these as thematic frames of analysis for our analytical departure point. We give them codes – real versus ideal, problems versus solutions, trust versus mistrust, co-production in action, the uniform, fiction versus non-fiction (there are only six, as some overlap).

Then we start analysing – only now it hits us that we're watching a video portrayal of a theatrical event in which "actors" are "real" people "acting" out their "real" experiences and perceptions of health and the health-care system. We're also watching ourselves in these scenes running around like researchers-cum-participant-observers-cum-"actors"-cum-intermediaries-between-organisational-"actors"-and-"community"-actors-cum-human-beings. We know these organisational actors as people who've tried to "help us" as BAMEs.

We know most of the other people from The Community as real people (BAMEs or otherwise), PIG people, research participants, and human beings.

We haven't applied for Ethics for this study but are piggybacking off the PIG Research Ethics Committee Ethics Approval XXX at XXX (redacted). We are interpreting our own data and experiences of reality, so that makes what we're doing ethical, particularly as we aren't using our own names. Although that throws up a few other ethical dilemmas.

If we aren't writing this, who is?

4.1.3 Sensemaking and meaning making

Our job here is meant to be relatively straightforward: to interpret the stories we see and hear in order to analyse the underlying narrative that we, as the storytellers, may not be able to give voice to ourselves (Riley and Hawe 2005).

But we've turned to the data for what feels like 10,000 hours and still there is no mastery of this analysis, though the interpretation (our "top line finding") seems glaringly obvious.[14]

Knowledge is power.

Whose knowledge matters? What knowledge counts?

These are our research questions.

We're beginning to realise we're welcomed as people who will bring "baseline" data to health improvement teams and public health, as long as the data arrives in the form that it needs to be in to be counted. A number. A curve on a graph. A clever quote in a questionnaire.

We don't belong to the organisation (NHS) but can really help them by giving our perceptions of health from minority ethnic groups living in a disadvantaged neighbourhood. So we are welcomed. When we go to PIG gatherings or Participatory Action Research (PAR) workshops or knowledge-exchange events like this one, we don't share the same language – "policy speak." We speak multiple other languages (English, Urdu, Slovak, Romanian, Polish, Other), but we might as well only speak one (the language of BAME).

We're no strangers to the polystyrene cups, freeze-dried coffee sachets, and mini milks that stand beside jugs of lukewarm water at PAR or PIG meetings. We're becoming familiar with most of the person-centred synonyms populating action plans and strategy documents and memos informed by conversations with people like us – actual human beings.

From a Community standpoint, we are welcomed as people who appear to be interested in actual human beings' lives, because these are the lives we are living. This is our reality. We sometimes don't belong to any of the ethnic groups "under investigation," but there's something about what we're doing and saying and what we look like that allows us to be received as BAMEs. As we're all in the same boat with this (some of us literally arrived here in boats – another story for another time), we are welcomed by each other (except when we are not).

When we catch up with other Community Members at local shops or events, we share the same language – "street speak." We're familiar with most of the challenges each person is telling the other when we chat in the corner shop or shisha café or library (even though we know we aren't supposed to be talking in libraries) so find some solidarity in that.

Okay, some of us look a bit similar, we'll give you that. Not entirely the same, but close enough to be different to the real natives. We also sound a bit (or very) different, depending on how long we've been here for, whether we're first, second, or third generation. If it's third generation, we sound completely native but still technically BAMEs.

Some of us had the necessary credentials to be researchers or doctors or dentists or lawyers in our countries, but not here. Here, we're BAMEs.

We suddenly remember we're writing an academic paper and think we should be quoting a scholar. Tom Stoppard. We know he's technically a playwright and screenwriter, but he was also a child refugee, and his work is peppered with humans rights themes – he's also a knight – so maybe citing him is acceptable: *"We are tied down to a language which makes up in obscurity what it lacks in style."*

This is a line from his absurdist, existentialist tragicomedy *Rosencrantz and Guildenstern Are Dead* (Stoppard 1966), in which the two lead characters spend the entire play in complete confusion, not even knowing their own identities. One of us first stumbled into the text during an undergraduate languages and literature course on *Intertextuality*. At that time, Anna was only interested in how the writing intersected with Shakespeare's *Hamlet* (in Polish), but has since discovered intertextuality is proper qualitative research method (it's been peer-reviewed and published!) for the analysis and interpretation of short narratives or life stories (Elkad-Lehman and Greensfeld 2011).

Had Anna been more focused in her late teens, she may have noticed that the life stories of Rosencrantz and Guildenstern were very complex but also very simple (not least because they were fictional). In the midst of existential crises, they could not make meaningful choices, and their lack of agency led to their death (in front of an audience).

4.1.4 Meaning in life, agency, and "choice"

We re-read the last few paragraphs, and just as we're about to delete them for being too tangential from our research questions – whose knowledge matters, what knowledge counts? – we spot some overarching themes: human rights, language, identity, methodology.

We also realise we've stumbled into the frames of analysis we'd originally sought to filter our research "data" through: real versus ideal, problems versus solutions, trust versus mistrust, co-production in action, the uniform, fiction versus nonfiction.

Let us try to explain. To address the research questions posed, we were originally going to present primary data in the "traditional way" from semi-structured interviews (n=35) with representatives from Community organisations and practitioners alongside organisational and Community ethnographies of the NHS and disadvantaged BAME groups respectively. Not that you have to quantify ethnographic observations, but we got to know sixty-four community members over six months (by co-existing within the same identity category [Box] in Hollow).

To shift towards a reflexive, critical view of "self," "other," and society in health research, we wanted to introduce creativity and relationality to our methodological approach. We wanted to present findings from the knowledge exchange project that transformed spectators – NHS practitioners, policymakers, Community Members, and third-sector organisations – by enabling them to step into, and change, the theatrical action presented by us, the performers (BAME and disadvantaged Community Members).

Come On In! used Theatre of the Oppressed techniques to breathe life into emotional and politicised findings gathered through ethnographies and interviews. The interactive performances starred us (Romanian Roma, Slovakian Roma, Pakistani, Polish, and other Community Members) and explored our (marginalised communities') perceptions of health and barriers to accessing services using an asset-based approach and co-production – bottom-up, community-driven approaches advocated by The State to address inequalities and facilitate rather than deliver public services.

Working with an experienced director, we (the Community Members) had a mechanism to express our perceptions – such as health research and community engagement being "tokenistic" and driven by the need to "tick a consultation box" – directly to practitioners and policymakers through a creative, non-threatening medium. Organisational actors (practitioners, policymakers, third-sector representatives) were then invited to enter scenes and alter them to encourage debate. This was not simply about reproducing reality or showing "role-play" situations in which there is a clear solution.

By using theatrical tools and "physicalising" subjective elements, the situations became much more "real" for all of us (participants) and revealed a palpable grittiness. You could see that the circumstances and issues enacted cannot be easily addressed through "surface-level" interventions that ignore structural problems. You could imagine how, if internalised, these circumstances and issues may perpetuate existential crises for individuals (us, you, others in the system).

Creativity opened up possible alternative scenarios so we could have a dialogue of knowledges (Freire 2005 [1972]) within the space. So all of us, as "spect-actors" (Boal 1985), could take off our masks to tell our "real" stories (through art). So all of us could put forward our perspectives to negotiating ways forward in a meaningful way.

For this to happen, we all had to want to be there. We all had to be ready to open up, unmask, and share. We had a full day of rehearsals in the community centre the day before the performance in the same venue in Hollow. There was space for twelve of us to take part. They said it wouldn't be possible to get twelve of us in one room at the same time and that none of us would arrive on time.

We all arrived. And we all arrived on time.

Three translators spoke Romanian, Slovakian, and Czech. We wanted more translators and in other languages, but this was the best they could do. On rehearsal day, we spoke about the researchers' findings and thought about what the results or problems might look like if they were in our bodies rather than on paper.

Then we created images and silent scenes to express them when words could only go so far. We presented this acting to fifty organisational actors the following day, and they were invited to come onstage at chosen moments of the drama (usually moments of tension or worry). They got to reimagine and remake these scenes by improvising with us.

4.1.5 *Real versus ideal*

Four people, a pram, and some chairs are in the (filmed) frame of the (staged) scene. The Community Members in this scene have some things in common – we all are "actors," we all are male, we all are "BAME." But we all sound different, look different, speak different languages, come in different shapes, shades, and sizes, wear different clothes, and have different roles.

We are acting out "real" (which we later turn to "ideal") images of our relationships with the NHS to a captive audience of "organisational-actors"-cum-"spect-actors."

"Three . . . two . . . one . . . go!" says the theatre director.

One of us instantly becomes hunched. He clutches his stomach and rubs it as he stumbles along with the aid of another person, who instantly reaches out to be his crutch. They hobble along together as two people watch. One has a wide smile on his face – he may be about to corpse. The other watches from his chair. He may just be sitting there (it isn't clear if he's actually meant to be in the scene).

As the limping pair lumbers along, we notice a fifth person (also male, also BAME) sitting next to the pram. Almost certainly not an "actor" – he's hiding his face in his jumper to stop him from laughing out loud. It's a silent scene so far. You hear someone (a "spect-actor") snigger.

The public health researcher animatedly runs into the scene and positions herself next to the pram, leaning in. It looks like she's trying to fit in with us. To belong.

There's an intrusive table with four chairs restaurant-style, but we're actually in a doctor's consulting room. A sixth person (female, BAME, "actor") gestures to a chair and whispers, "Please." The companion helps the sick man with stomach problems into a chair. They sit squarely before a serious-looking seventh person (male, BAME, "actor"), while the sixth person shuffles some paperwork.

"What's your name?"

A soft, inaudible sound.

"What's your name?"

The same again, but she clearly hears it this time as she starts going through a list of names on her blank sheet of paper.

"No appointment, sorry." She gestures to where they came from (imagine a door). The companion becomes instantly incensed.

"This the problem!" he says in a raised voice, pointing at person number 1. "This the problem!"

The sick man repeats, "Problem!" He clutches his stomach. "Sorry, sorry, problem!"

A chorus of "Sorries!" and "Problems!"

The sixth person is having none of this. She pushes him towards the (imagined) door. "Go, go, go!"

They all speak over one another so you can't really make out the rest of the words, but you can tell it isn't good. In the background, you can hear the translator decoding.

The sick man clasps his stomach as the companion helps him to the (imagined) door. Then he raises his arms as if to indicate applause. The director goes "Woop!" then everybody claps. The "actors" smile and applaud themselves. Only forty-six seconds have passed.

The camera zooms out to reveal a captive audience of "community actors," which includes another pram (this one with a baby in it). We have to bring our children to rehearsals and performances as paying for childcare isn't an option. Most of us don't have jobs.

This scene ("not having an appointment") is one of three showing a barrier in accessing health services for us. The other two ("no National Insurance number" and "wrong interpreter") are performed to "organisational actors," and we discuss how these barriers could be removed.

What could be done differently?

4.1.6 Problems versus solutions

"The way that the man was dealing with them, there was nothing personal about it. There was no eye contact. It was just 'number, number, number, out.' No interaction. No smiles. No anything to make them feel comfortable."

We can hear the translator frantically interpreting this "organisational actor's" observation. A "community actor" walks in front of the camera, carrying her baby. She plants a kiss on her cheek just as the director asks the same "organisational actor," "So what can you do, then, to make them feel more comfortable?"

Two additional people appear in the frame. They are female "spect-actors," just like the twelve people behind them, but they are wearing headscarves.

"Eye contact. Smile."

"Can I just stop you there? Can you just show me, very quickly?"

We all erupt into spontaneous applause as the "spect-actor" takes to the stage to rearrange the now-improvised scene.

"Three . . . two . . . one . . . go!"

Just as the "organisational actor" assumes her role as receptionist in the doctor's consulting room (she is carrying the blank sheets of paper and a pen), a young child runs in front of her (the son of a "community actor" who isn't in the scene). We all laugh at the intrusion. Suddenly the scene seems more human even though it remains unchanged.

"Hi, how are you?"

The "organisational actor" looks the first of five "community actors" sitting in a queue, waiting to see the doctor, while clutching her (actual) child (a "spect-actor" for the purposes of this scene).

"Fine."

"Do you have the information? Your National Insurance number?"

She does. There's an exchanging of papers. A "Thank you very much," then on to the next person.

"Good morning, how are you?"

The second "community actor," wearing a stripy top, nods from side to side as if to say, "Okay."

"Okay." The paperwork in order, the "organisation actor" moves on to the third person, wearing a pink headscarf. All smiles. There appear to be no problems here.

"Thank you very much." Then on to the next "community actor," wearing a black headscarf.

"Good morning, hi." The translator exchanges the pleasantries.

"Good morning, how are you?"

Through the translator we hear that the fifth "community actor" is quite sick and waiting to be seen by a doctor. He doesn't have a National Insurance number.

This was the moment of discontent when the scene was first enacted, and all eyes are on the "organisational actor" as she responds, "Okay, if you can possible please hang on for about five or ten minutes, I'll be able to find out the information about how you can get your NI number, and then I'll get back to you. Is that okay with you?"

He is nodding and smiling, so we think this is okay with him.

"Right, thank you." There is more smiling and nodding, by the "organisational actor" this time. We think everything is going to be okay here.

"Woop!"

It's the end of the scene, and we all applaud and cheer.

We drop our masks as "spect-actors," and in the ensuing discussion, the Community Member who played the fifth "community actor" explains why the re-enacted alternative felt like progress even though he didn't have an NI: "Perfect won't exist anywhere, but better can exist."

4.1.7 Trust versus mistrust

Flash forward to the next series of scenes in which we, "community actors," are embodying our "mistrust" of health-care organisations. A queue of people waits to see the doctor. One finally manages to see him, but when the doctor is presented with medical tests from a different country, she is told to go away. He can't accept them. The others wait in line, silently.

The director goes 'round, tapping each "community actor" on the shoulder. They each, in turn, say one line to voice (through an interpreter) what they're thinking right now.

Tap. "I've been waiting for three hours. I can't do this anymore." A female in a bright-yellow jumper with a red-and-white headscarf.

Tap. "We're waiting, and nobody's talking to us to even tell us anything." A female in a red jumper with a black headscarf.

Tap. "I'm hungry." A male holding a newspaper.

Quite a few of us are permanently hungry as we roam the streets. We've seen people like you look at us sideways as we've scraped through bins, looking for scraps of food, and let our children steal apples from the grocer as they walk past.

It's easy to judge. You might do the same if you were us.

"Community actors" are granted three wishes to help us improve those scenes. There's a scurry of activities in ten seconds, then the director yells, "Freeze!"

"Audience, what changes have they made?"

"Community actors" respond in unison. "Smiling." "Smiling helps with trust." "Eye contact." "Everyone with a happier face that's appreciative of the better situation they are in."

Perhaps our data has reached the point of saturation?

We flick through the feedback forms from *Come On In!* One "organisational actor" writes:

> "We can all work better and more compassionately with service users no matter what their nationality is – some of the scenarios depicted what many indigenous people experience as well as diverse communities."

4.1.8 Lunch: the finger food situation

In the middle of all this acting, it's lunchtime, and we stop for refuelling. We, "community actors," do the thing we did during rehearsal day. Tables, crushed against the walls to maximise stage floor space, are carried into the centre of the community centre hall and set up to look like a head table at a wedding party.

We pile mini crustless triangles and fists full of crisps onto one plate to feed one family. We put the plate in the middle so everyone can share. There's no "my plate" or "your plate." My "sandwich" or your "samosa." There's just food for sharing. Food for feeding. And we talk and we laugh as our little ones run around and take more food so there's less for the big ones. There's noise. There's life. One of us starts playing the accordion.

This is how we eat. This is how we live.

We look beyond our top table to the sides of the hall, where most "organisational actors" stand alone or in packs of two or three. Paper plates in one hand, phones in the other. They aren't talking to each other. Looks like they're working hard. Everything they do must be urgent. They must have things to do ASAP!

4.2 Discussion

We haven't followed the "right" structure for this peer-reviewed paper. Our multiple methods have been mad. A methodological mess.

We're guessing our knowledge won't matter here. Our knowledge won't count.

We've tried to use thematic coding to structure our findings and feelings, but this all feels a bit forced. We'd rather sing or cook or make music or speak to you about our lives than put it in a [Box] or write about it. We don't always want to write things down. Some of us can't write. Some of us can't write in this language. Some of us are professional post-graduates in our countries.

Some of us would rather feel our way through our experiences – or find a way to escape them – but you make us think about it and talk about it. We'd rather not be in touch with everything that is real about our "reality."

We cannot give you *an answer*. We cannot give you *the answer*. We are not homogenous. We do not identify as BAME or any of the other categories you have given us to pick.

If you want to co-produce a health service with us to improve our health outcomes, let's call it The Void. You'll need to figure out how to see, touch, or measure the essence of us. The essence of you. The essence of you and us relating, creatively, experiencing reality together.

***

INTERLUDE – CONNECTING THE INDIVIDUAL TO THE SYSTEM

It's been almost a decade since I read Nancy Krieger's seminal paper *"Who and what is a 'population'?"* The social epidemiologist got me thinking about how to connect the individual to the system. How to make the system more human. How to think of public health as a discipline that needs to think about personal encounters that can't be generalised alongside broader perspectives at a population level.

Nancy notes that "'population' and 'individual' are not antonyms," but rather on a spectrum of belonging with "individuum" being on the one end as "the smallest unit" with characteristics of the "whole" to which it inherently belongs (Williams 1985). The "reality" is that the individual and population exist and experience life "simultaneously" as both a person (singular) and a person who's part of a population (collectively). "This joint fact," Nancy says, "is fundamental and is essential to keep in mind if analysis of either individual or population phenomena is to be valid" (Krieger 2012).[15]

Nancy truly troubled the notion of causality in sciences by putting "the idea and reality of 'population'" under the microscope. Sure, you can generalise, aggregate, correlate, and calculate the statistical mean of any given population, but whether you end up with any sort of meaningful data will depend on understanding the *relationships* between individuals within that defined population and also outside the "group." In other words, "populations are dynamic beings constituted by intrinsic relationships both among their members and with the other populations that together produce their existence and make meaningful casual inference possible."[16]

I think about the injustices I may have inadvertently perpetuated by "forcing" the mentally "unwell," "disabled" (Deaf), "disadvantaged," and BAME populations into a category-framework-identity they didn't "fit into."

To what extent did their knowledge – in its "truest" expression – really matter to the public health system?

To what extent did measuring their experiences make any difference to their actual lived experiences?

In one of my studies – while we made music and danced and ate and were merry in a community centre – "BAME (Roma)" participants linked racism to poor health outcomes and explained how they hid their identities as Gypsies out of fear of being discriminated against.

To what extent could any public health intervention improve this population's health, then, unless there is a seismic attempt to tackle "structural racism"?[17]

According to Zinzi D Bailey, Nancy Krieger, and others writing in *The Lancet*,

> The stark reality is that research investigating the relationship between structural racism and population health outcomes has been scant, and even less work has been done to assess the health impacts of the few interventions and policy changes that could help dismantle structural racism.

Dismantling structural determinants of health through a public health intervention.

Where would we even begin?

I think of In-Credible sitting around a fake fire in a fake forest on top of a fake building in a fake disadvantaged neighbourhood inspired by real community members' stories of their real-life experiences as they've taken part in real research to inform public health interventions.

How would they stage an intervention?

***

Notes

1 Here's the soundtrack to this scene from Behind the Noise: Stream "Tell Me" by Half Life Human (Cleveden Secondary School) by Behind the Noise | Listen online for free on SoundCloud. https://soundcloud.com/behindthenoise/tell-me-by-half-life-human-cleveden-secondary-27219
2 Direct quotes are lyrics taken from "Tell Me" by "Half Life Human", as earlier.
3 An influential term coined by anthropologist Clifford Geertz, "thick description" captures more than human behaviour but offers an explanation of it within its context to make it more meaningful to outsiders (Geertz 1973). A "granular ethnography" attends to the complexities of daily social life in its theorising and methodology (Atkinson 2017).
4 Page 1.
5 Page 143.
6 Page 13.
7 Page 46.
8 Page 44.
9 Page 66.
10 Page 46.
11 Michel Foucault's unique connection of power and knowledge gets us thinking about how the two concepts are interrelated and "speak" to each other. Jackson and Mazzei use this to dig deep into "manifestations of power/knowledge" in practices as individuals within institutions "negotiate power relations and new knowledge about themselves," thereby "disrupt[ing] historical truths or struggle[s]" (Jackson and Mazzei 2017) (page 57).
12 I'd been brewing over and writing about this concept for six years, ever since the Theatre of the Oppressed study with marginalised groups that you're about to become familiar with (de Andrade 2016). Then, a few months ago, I stumbled into Rachel Horst's paper on "Narrative Futuring," which really resonated with it. The PhD student of Language and Literacy Education similarly "invite[s] the unruly, the irreverent, and the absurd" into her experimental writing, positing "future fiction as research." Drawing on Bruner's (1991) notion that narrative "operates as an instrument of mind in the construction of reality," Rachel asserts that "the personal, the fanciful, the theoretical, and the absurd are intentionally entangled, commingled, and co-productive" in her writing-researching (Horst 2021).
13 (Barthes 1971) cited by Krause-Jensen on page 23 of *Flexible Firm: The Design of Culture at Bang & Olufsen* (Krause-Jensen 2010).
14 In his book *Outliers*, journalist Malcolm Gladwell says it takes roughly ten thousand hours of practice to achieve mastery in a field (Gladwell 2008).
15 Page 651.
16 Pages 636–37.
17 *Structural racism* refers to "the totality of ways in which societies foster [racial] discrimination, via mutually reinforcing [inequitable] systems. . . (e.g., in housing, education, employment, earnings, benefits, credit, media, health care, criminal justice, etc.) that in turn reinforce discriminatory beliefs, values, and distribution of resources," reflected in history, culture, and interconnected institutions (Bailey et al. 2017) (page 1).

References

Arva, Eugene L. 2008. "Writing the Vanishing Real: Hyperreality and Magical Realism." *JNT-Journal of Narrative Theory* 38 (1): 60–85. https://doi.org/10.1353/JNT.0.0002.

Atkinson, Paul. 2017. *Thinking Ethnographically*. 1st ed. London: SAGE Publications Ltd.

Bailey, Zinzi D., Nancy Krieger, Madina Agénor, Jasmine Graves, Natalia Linos, and Mary T. Bassett. 2017. "Structural Racism and Health Inequities in the USA: Evidence and Interventions." *The Lancet* 389 (10077): 1453–63. https://doi.org/10.1016/S0140-6736(17)30569-X.

Barthes, Roland. 1971. *Ecrivains, Intellectuels, Professeurs*. du Seuil. https://books.google. co.uk/books/about/Ecrivains_intellectuels_professeurs.html?id=xLsjnwEACAAJ &redir_esc=y.

Boal, Augusto. 1985. *Theatre of the Oppressed*. New York: Theatre Communications Group.

Bruner, Jerome. 1991. *The Narrative Construction of Reality. Critical Inquiry*. 1st ed. Vol. 18. University of Chicago Press. www.jstor.org/stable/1343711.

de Andrade, Marisa de. 2016. "The Masks We Wear and Stories We Tell in Organisations: Exploring How Spirituality and Creativity Can Provide Purpose and Reduce 'Othering.'" In *11th Organization Studies Summer Workshop on Spirituality, Symbolism, and Storytelling*, edited by G. Balint, B. Antala, C. Carty, J-M. A. Mabieme, I. B. Amar, and A. Kaplanova, 343–54. Mykonos: Greece. https://doi.org/10.2/JQUERY.MIN.JS.

Deleuze, Gilles, and Félix Guattari. 2000. *Anti-Oedipus. Capitalism and Schizophrenia*. Minneapolis: University of Minnesota Press.

Elkad-Lehman, Ilana, and Hava Greensfeld. 2011. "Intertextuality as an Interpretative Method in Qualitative Research." *Narrative Inquiry* 21 (2): 258–75. https://doi. org/10.1075/NI.21.2.05ELK/CITE/REFWORKS.

Freire, Paulo. 2005 [1972]. *Pedagogy of the Oppressed: 30th Anniversary Edition*. New York: The Continuum International Publishing Group Inc.

Gale, Ken. 2018. *Madness as Methodology: Bringing Concepts to Life in Contemporary Theorising and Inquiry*. New York: Routledge.

Geertz, Clifford. 1973. *Thick Description: Toward an Interpretive Theory of Culture*. New York, NY: Basic Book.

Gladwell, Malcolm. 2008. *Outliers*. New York: Little, Brown and Company.

Horst, Rachel. 2021. "Narrative Futuring: An Experimental Writing Inquiry Into the Future Imaginaries." *Art/Research International* 6 (1). https://journals.library.ualberta.ca/ ari/index.php/ari/article/view/29554/22016.

Jackson, Alecia Youngblood, and Lisa A. Mazzei. 2017. "Thinking with Theory: A New Analytic for Qualitative Inquiry." In *The SAGE Handbook of Qualitative Research*, 717–37. SAGE Publications Inc.

Krause-Jensen, Jakob. 2010. *Flexible Firm : The Design of Culture at Bang & Olufsen*. New York: Berghahn Books, Inc.

Krieger, Nancy. 2012. "Who and What Is a 'Population'? Historical Debates, Current Controversies, and Implications for Understanding 'Population Health' and Rectifying Health Inequities." *The Milbank Quarterly* 90 (4): 634–81. https://doi. org/10.1111/J.1468-0009.2012.00678.X.

Riley, Therese, and Penelope Hawe. 2005. "Researching Practice: The Methodological Case for Narrative Inquiry." *Health Education Research* 20 (2): 226–36. https://doi. org/10.1093/HER/CYG122.

Stoppard, Tom. 1966. *Rosencrantz and Guildenstern Are Dead*. London: Faber and Faber.

Whitehead, Alfred North. 1929. *Process and Reality. An Essay in Cosmology, Gifford Lectures Delivered in the University of Edinburgh During the Session 1927–28*. Cambridge, UK: Cambridge University Press.

Williams, Raymond. 1985. *Keywords: A Vocabulary of Culture and Society*. New York: Oxford University Press.

5 Can you hear me?

We re-join In-Credible, Sara, and sixty-four Community Members sitting around a flickering fire in the majestic Futile Forest on the 212th floor of the infamous Beguile Building, shaped like a ginormous bulbous pear.

The daybreak would be peeking out if the sun weren't hiding behind thick clouds with a red exclamation mark on the weather forecast. "Warnings Issued," says the triangle alert on the Flower Supermoon one day in May in The Future. It's two degrees Celsius, and gloveless fingers are being bitten by an unforgiving windchill.

In-Credible looks troubled as she reflects on all that has happened since she first saw Sara through the windscreen of her terrestrial e-Charge as it cruised towards high-rises just a few hours earlier.

"I was in charge of this story," she tells the Community Members as one of them (the long Deaf one who didn't ignore Sara in the toilet) goes around pouring everyone a cup of hot cacao from a silver flask. "I was the one with the rigorous research design, with the data, with the framework, with the ethics approval, with the insight. I was writing this story in the first person at the start of this book . . ." She stops to take a sip of thick bitterness. "Now I'm not even the storyteller anymore. Someone is speaking on my behalf. Where have 'I' gone?"

"Welcome to our world," Lena says, speaking through an interpreter, rolling her eyes.

"I don't know why you're being so precious," Anna says through a Polish interpreter. "Haven't you heard of Judith Butler?"

"You've heard of Judith Butler?"

"You're so surprised someone like me from somewhere that isn't here might have studied someone like Judith at a University in my own country? Or come across her on the internet . . . the same internet that you use?"

"That's not what I meant . . ."

That's exactly what she meant.

"You see, who is that person writing now? It isn't me. It isn't Sara. Who are you?" In-Credible looks up to the heavens.

It's me. Marisa. No need to look up, In-Credible. I'm not playing God here. I'm human. I'm with you – right there – knowing-telling-showing what it is you're

DOI: 10.4324/9781003196488-5

experiencing (Richardson and St Pierre 2005).[1] *Now stop being so incredulous and listen to what Anna's got to say about Judith Butler . . .*

"In speaking the 'I,' I undergo something of what cannot be captured or assimilated by the 'I,' since I always arrive too late to myself," (Butler 2001)[2] quotes Anna.

But In-Credible doesn't want to let this go.

"Marisa," she says, still sipping cacao, "you don't even belong here with all these made-up characters. You should be in the other parallel part of this book with all the academic references. What are you calling those sections – interludes?"

I don't know if I'm calling them interludes yet. Maybe. I'm still working on it.

"Well, you better get your skates on. Your book's due to the publisher in three weeks."

Thanks for the reminder, In-Credible. Time moves forward; it never moves back. If you stopped worrying so much about arriving at the "end" with your fixed findings and conclusions and recommendations and just tried to "be with" the theory right now as you try to make sense of your data, you might realise that your identity crisis is very much part of the process . . .

"What do you mean?"

Well, I'm thinking that this is what researchers in public health do. We create distance. Separate ourselves from the person we're trying to connect with as if there's you (me-I) and them (other). As if the empirical, analytical space between the two produces "real" knowledge rather than using that gap to produce new knowledge. Maybe think of the "I" as "a mangle composed of multiple elements." How we define that "mangle" in a "social script" is one way of making sense of it, but there are other ways too. That "mangle" has "a body that is sexed and raced, a body that is located at a particular place in the social hierarchy, and a body/subject that has had a range of experiences." Maybe this means the "I" fits nicely within the confines of the "social script" attributed to it. But maybe it doesn't fit at all. "In all cases," though, "there is no single causal factor determining the subject; the elements of subjectivity intra-act in a complex web" (Hekman 2010).[3]

"What are you trying to say?" In-Credible asks. She's getting shifty. Troubled. "I came here to make sense of the SILLY Clinical Trial data, to analyse this collective psychosis in The Community, and here I am . . . hours later . . . what time is it . . . ?"

"Time's just a construct," chides Anna.

"Enough already! Here I am on this random rooftop, no further forward . . . . What am I supposed to report back to Professor Ebba? How am I supposed to make sense of what is real . . . scientific, objective, valid . . . true? And what is unreal . . . fiction, subjective, opinion . . . made up?" Her hands cover her face, as if she's playing peek-a-boo with a toddler.

Sara materialises as if she's been there all along. As if someone – me, Marisa, I'm guessing – has just drawn her into the scene like a sketch on a blank canvas.

She nudges In-Credible, who peeps at Sara through her fingers.

"What have you got in your hand?"

Angels chant a virtuous anthem of doom in unison as a miracle appears in In-Credible's hand – Sara's little black pouch. The one with the seventeen one-terabyte memory sticks.

"Memory sticks?" In-Credible asks, incredulously (there are other adverbs, but this one works too well here, so worthy of the repetition, I think).

"Your data," Sara says as Mark Rodger takes the sticks from her, "we're staging an intervention."

"Plug it in,[4] Kelvin," Mark says to a teenager speaking through a British Sign Language (BSL) interpreter.

"Hey, hang on, is that a kid? Do we have ethics for this?" In-Credible asks.

> *Relax. Of course the study has ethical approval. He's from Behind the Noise.*
> *He belongs here . . .*

The sensor-synchronised 4DX screens surrounding them become a giant desktop. In-Credible's encrypted data pops up on the screen in separate folders, one for each study.

"How did you get into that? It's password-protected." In-Credible stares at the monitor as reams and reams of raw data burst from the dossiers.

"Turn that off!" she shouts, jumping up and down, her arms waving about as she tries to cover up the information, but to no avail. She's a silhouetted ant on a colossal projection. "I haven't anonymised- or pseudonymised-removed identifying characteristics from the dataset yet!"

> *You've tried that, actually, In-Credible. Anonymity and pseudonymisation wasn't*
> *an option, remember? You've coded data to obscurity, and even still it's blindingly*
> *obvious who the participants are due to the nature of this data. You're just going to*
> *have to trust in the process . . .*

"What process?"

Anna arrives on the scene. She's reading out loud from a hardcover copy of *Thinking with Theory in Qualitative Research: Viewing Data Across Multiple Perspectives*:

> *Certainly what we envisioned for this project was not grounded in traditional coding*
> *and thematic, conventional analysis of data, with emphasis on the production of an*
> *end or commodity. Rather, we positioned our project as a production of knowledge*
> *that might emerge as a creation out of chaos. Coding and data reduction then would*
> *be seen as commodification and the process of plugging in as a production of the new,*
> *the assemblage in formation. Imagine this production of knowledge – emerging as*
> *assemblage, creation from chaos – not as a final arrival, but as the result of plugging*
> *in: an assemblage of "continuous, self-vibrating intensities" that required discarding*

the tripartite division between a field of reality (the world) and a field of representation (the book) and a field of subjectivity (the author). Rather, an assemblage establishes connections between certain multiplicities drawn from each of these orders, so that a book has no sequel nor the world as its object nor one or several authors as its subject.
(Jackson and Mazzei 2012)[5]

"Wow . . . too much information to process.

  Too short a space of time.

We're such badly built machines.
  We humans.
  We think we're so smart and sophisticated, but we're full of flaws. Layer
                upon layer
      upon layer
of unprocessed thoughts and memories and nightmares.
      And dreams.
  All just accumulating.   Amounting to nothing."
Mark and Kelvin take their places on either side of the virtual desktop. A song by the Attention Seekers from Behind the Noise[6] fills the frosty air, softly at first, then bellowing:

  "Did she help you move on in the real world?
  I've been dreaming of another universe, where you get everything you want . . .
  And everything is perfect . . ."[7]
  "You're going to have to start feeling again, In-Credible," Sara says as sparks fly in the sky.

Bright white veins pierce the thick blanket of black clouds. Somewhere in the cosmos, hot air meets cold air. A crack of thunder drowns out the music to welcome the downpour.

***

INTERLUDE – BREATHING LIFE INTO PUBLIC HEALTH DATA AND EVALUATION USING CREATIVE-RELATIONAL INQUIRY

ROUTLEDGE BOOK PROPOSAL

CHAPTER ABSTRACT

5. Can you hear me?

  The Deaf Community Comedy Cult meets Behind the Noise one rainy Wednesday afternoon (why is it always raining?) in the basement of a pub in Hollow with members of The Mainstream (people who don't have a disability). Their leader, renowned and controversial, goes by the unassuming name of John Smith[8] (truth; you couldn't make this up). For today's gathering, he's brought a bag of sensory instruments – such as magnifying glasses to see better and megaphones to amplify voices to hear better – as the word on the street is that The Mainstream has recently reported an inability to feel (ironically making them "disabled," too, but never mind). Disconnected from their senses, they are sleepwalking through life, intellectualising each encounter; more and more of them are developing mental health problems.

Public health experts (from The Mainstream), who were brought in to investigate this phenomenon, produced and analysed big datasets at breakneck speed. Then they hit a wall. It's an oddity. They simply cannot make sense of their findings using rationality, reasoning, and logic.

The Deaf Community Comedy Cult and Behind the Noise decide it is time to stage an *intervention*, which, paradoxically, involves critiquing public health and community *interventions*, evaluations, and the evidence that feed in to them. Equipped with theories of embodiment, trauma, psychoanalysis, and relational ethics, they bring emotion back in to the business of public health research, policy, and practice. They also introduce comedy and music as methodology to public health.

This story merges two framework applications. Firstly, the author's NHS Greater Glasgow and Clyde project exploring the value of people's stories and experiences expressed through the medium of comedy. It aimed to break down barriers and co-produce appropriate services with the Deaf Community and mental health professionals. It also sought to shape local action plans and legislation, particularly in relation to the British Sign Language (BSL) Act; establish unmet needs of BSL users in relation to mental health; improve Deaf people's knowledge of mental health services; and establish Best Practice in mental health services and prevention for BSL users.

Secondly, a collaboration with the project Behind the Noise (BTN), an award-winning and accredited music and skills programme funded by an Economic and Social Research Council (ESRC) Impact Accelerator Account and Knowledge and Impact grants from the University of Edinburgh's College of Arts Humanities and Social Sciences (CAHSS). *Measuring Humanity through Music in Schools* applied the framework in secondary mainstream and assisted learning schools in areas of multiple deprivation.

When trying to get an academic book commissioned, you have to give specialists in your field the right amount of information on which to judge the quality of your work.[9] I wrote the previous abstract for Chapter 5 in the proposal I submitted to Routledge to help them and reviewers judge this book's suitability for publication.

I knew I wanted to write a story like this, but organising your thoughts and chapters in such a linear way isn't particularly straightforward when using humanities and arts-informed, post-qualitative methodologies. It's difficult to know from the onset where the inquiry begins and where it ends.

If I'm thinking with Ken Gale, who's thinking with Erin Manning, who's thinking with Simondon:

> I am not necessarily intending to offer starting points or places where this book and these ideas of methodology . . . somehow began to emerge and form as part of some kind of linear process which had a beginning, in the past tense, is being presented here and now in some kind of present and will have an ending in some kind of future.
>
> (Gale 2018)[10]

I think about what this means in relation to Measuring Humanity, the programme of research that got me writing this book in the first place. My intentions were "pure," but my analysis constrained through the formulation of a framework that I-we-they (researcher-academy-funder-policymaker) believed we needed for the research to be credible.

I had a nagging feeling all along that I needed to take a deep dive into the data – to be "inside of the credible datasets" (in-Credible) – to touch the essence of what was happening when I connected with humans in this way (or as much as you can touch the essence of humanity through the written word). Then, when I "plugged in" creative-relational inquiry into the framework, something cracked open.

Writing with Jonathan Wyatt and Rosie Stenhouse, the director and another associate director for the Centre for Creative-Relational Inquiry, we "problematized and provided alternatives for, taken-for-granted assumptions concerning research and research practices" (de Andrade, Stenhouse, and Wyatt 2020):[11]

JONATHAN: Take it to heart. Massumi suggests the creative-relational is a process of becoming, with desire as its force. Creative-relational inquiry is concept, not methodology. It's inquiry that seeks not to "capture" and hold still, but to find a way, through desire, to do justice to the fluidity of process.

MARISA: There are different ways of knowing, so why is my knowing as a "public health elite" more than the knowing of the marginalized community members I engage with, dance with, make theatre with, make art with? Why are bodies, dissenting voices, hearts, excluded from an evidence-base that accepts only the written word and manipulated numbers – coded, aggregated – as evidence? . . . My sense is that public health researchers need to take their work to heart. Feel the beating of our hearts as we gather and analyse data. Be affected by blood-pumping, heart-racing, flip-flopping, head-over-heel moments of connection in the field and at our desks, rather than putting emotions aside as we make sense of big data. Ignoring each heart palpitation, as we work on aggregation . . . public health problems are persisting – exacerbating – despite significant policy and research investments. Poor health, pervasive inequalities, untenable pressure on health and social care services. Everything we've tried hasn't worked. Why not try something radically different?

How to move from reductionism to interpretivism to "methodology against interpretivism" (Jackson and Mazzei 2013) – or something radically different – in public health to produce more meaningful insights?

Guided by Alecia Jackson and Lisa Mazzei's pivotal text, I began thinking about what would happen if I moved away from thematic coding and an iterative approach to meaning-making to "thinking with theory and plugging one text into another." How could this "open up" latent knowledge in the datasets and "proliferate rather than foreclose and simplify findings?" (Jackson and Mazzei 2013).[12]

My methodological approach and writing style shifted significantly as I put this alternative thinking to work. As I moved from an emotionally disconnected, flat, objective analysis that left me wanting to know more to an immersive, embodied, creative-relational inquiry.

My journey began with "traditional" abduction. Here's how it started – in the straitjacket of traditional public health methodologies and structured writing.

5.1 Thinking with abduction

5.1.1 Introduction

Emotional well-being has several benefits associated with health, relationships, and life chances and is a key area of research in public health interventions and policies (Kobau et al. 2011; National Institute for Health and Care Excellence 2012). Recent advancements in neuroscience, however, have produced compelling evidence against our classical understanding of emotions as "built in," "universal," and comprised of emotion circuits in our brains causing a discrete set of changes to the human experience. The theory of constructed emotion questions the existence of emotion "fingerprints" with objective criteria to accurately measure emotion. Instead, "emotional granularity" proposes that emotions vary considerably from person to person and between cultures and are products of social reality rather than being real in the objective sense (Barrett 2017).[13]

This has wide-ranging implications for population health research, evaluation, practice, and policy – particularly when investigating health inequalities – as public health is largely informed by categorisation, essentialism, and reductionism of demographic groups and emotions (Ellison 2010). There is little research on how our experience of an emotion or feeling impacts and contributes to our health behaviours and decision-making (Ferrer and Mendes 2018). Furthermore, what we know is largely informed by changes in self-reported measures or observable expressions of specific conceptualisations of emotions that affect mental and physical health (Ciuk, Troy, and Jones 2015). Evaluations of interventions, policies, and practices based on datasets of categorised emotions could therefore be misleading if reanalysed through this theoretical lens.

This writing reflects on what novel insights might emerge by bringing contemporary neuroscience theory to public health to investigate emotions – how they are conceptualised, understood, experienced, and expressed by community members, particularly in marginalised groups – in the context of gathering evidence for and from population health interventions. Specifically, it seeks to understand how categorising emotions at the population level enables or hinders intervention implementation and evaluation, and how this impacts policy and practice.

A multiple-case-study-replication approach informed by health humanities and arts is used to investigate the study's underlying theoretical proposition – that we can work with community members to identify and categorise attributes, including emotions and outcomes, that maximise their health and well-being. To facilitate this inquiry, a co-produced methodological evaluation framework (or Asset-Based Indicator Framework) is applied in various settings with different communities to measure impacts of creative community engagement on emotions linked to health.

The writing begins with a background on the design, implementation, and evaluation of complex public health interventions. The focus is on what evidence is used in this process and how emotions feature. The next section explains how applying the Asset-Based Indicator Framework (also called the Framework) in various settings provides a mechanism to establish distinct emotion categories for specific communities that lead to context-specific conceptualisations of health and aspects related to well-being.

The methodological section details the multiple-case-study design with the initial step of theory development and the selection of five cases examining emotional experiences of marginalised groups through creative community engagements: self-identified Gypsies engaging through music; community members in disadvantaged neighbourhoods using a range of creative activities; the Deaf community using comedy; community members at risk of poor mental health engaged in green spaces and environmental art activities; and school pupils from areas of multiple deprivation producing and performing original music.

A two-step analytical procedure is employed, firstly by applying the Framework to individual cases. A cross-case thematic analysis follows. Findings are critically analysed under key themes: self-reported emotions; same emotion, different emotional experience; subjective personal experiences, trauma, and the system; and creative interventions for emotion regulation and coping. The discussion then considers findings through the lens of the theory of constructed emotion, thereby challenging key public health conventions on the design, implementation, and evaluation of complex interventions. Important implications for international research, policy, and practice are presented in the conclusion.

5.1.2 Measuring emotions in complex systems

A complex adaptive systems approach challenges simple cause-and-effect assumptions by considering how different parts of the system interact and relate, thereby affecting and being shaped by the system (The Health Foundation 2010). Various parts adapt by changing together – influencing one another and their context – so these are essentially living systems comprised of free individual agents acting unpredictably (Plsek and Wilson 2001).

Human traits, such as varying emotional experiences, present an element of vagueness when developing and evaluating interventions in these systems. Political and socio-economic determinants of health add to the complexity, particularly when investigating wicked issues – multifaceted problems with multiple possible causes; internal, nonlinear dynamics; and detrimental societal consequences if unaddressed (Peters 2017). Examples include poverty, equality, and well-being. There is no one-size-fits-all solution for these issues, so replicability is not only challenging but could also potentially exacerbate public health problems (Greenhalgh and Papoutsi 2018).

Researchers, funders, practitioners, and policymakers are grappling with how to validate and evaluate public health interventions in complex systems. A basis is to make use of theory before testing and to integrate theoretical insights into an explicit model of how an intervention could change behaviour or affect other connections in the causal chain between intervention and outcome (Craig 2006). The value of this causal modelling approach is the choice of intervention points and associated measures along the causal pathway that can be used for evaluation.

Measurement, however, has become a contentious issue in population health with measures, markers, and evidence generally conceptualised through positivist approaches valuing the scientific method in knowledge generation rather than how people feel (de Andrade and Angelova 2020). These approaches conflict with principles of co-production that involve rich understandings of the lived experience of a person, who is meant to play an equal and active role in determining their own outcomes (Loeffler et al. 2013). Indeed, guidance from funders on the development, evaluation, and implementation of complex interventions to improve health has noted that subjective or self-reported outcomes may be erroneous, particularly if the study is unblinded (Craig 2006).

When community members' feelings are taken into account in public health interventions and evaluations, they tend to be assessed quantitatively through "validated" psychosocial measurement scales that may also produce misleading data when contextualised (de Andrade and Angelova 2020; Shavers 2007).

A person's experience of a feeling or emotion is an internal process. We therefore rely on self-reported or observable expressions of emotion based on our own interpretations of a person's emotional experience through the ways in which they express their emotions or feelings. In health assessments and evaluations informed by the emotion-health relationship, we are also guided by how one's feelings or emotions are revealed to others through language, voice tone, body language, facial expressions, and visible signs of emotion, such as tears, laughter, or frowns (Barrett 2016).

Capturing emotion-health changes at the community level is even more challenging due to variations within and across population groups. However, we need an understanding of how different populations account for emotional attributes in relation to their well-being to know whether population-level interventions measuring changes in emotional well-being – linked to physical and mental health – lead to improved health outcomes.

Attempts to evaluate these approaches have leaned on realistic evaluations, theories of change, and logic modelling but fallen short of providing a systematic way of capturing changes in "softer" emotional outcomes (such as trust and happiness) at the community level linked to health, well-being, and inequalities (see Public Health England for a summary of tested community-centred approaches and evidence).[14]

5.1.3 Methods

A co-produced methodological evaluation framework – Asset-Based Indicator Framework – was therefore developed and piloted with Black Minority Ethnic groups. It provides a mechanism to establish distinct emotion categories for specific communities that are linked to community-defined conceptualisations of health and well-being; co-produce health outcomes that are meaningful for specific populations; and identify actions to inform improved policy and practice for particular groups. If co-produced with a marginalised community, the Framework also helps us understand the reasons underpinning inequality for that particular community at individual, community, and structural levels (de Andrade and Angelova 2020).

In this writing, the Framework is applied across five case studies to identify and categorise attributes and emotions linked to health and well-being in distinct community settings. As the aim was to understand how emotions are conceptualised, understood, experienced, and expressed by community members in different marginalised groups, a multiple-case-study approach was well suited to capture context-specific perceptions within each community setting and across settings (Abma and Stake 2014).

The theory-first approach of multiple-case-replication design guides data collection and analysis (Yin 2014). A key theoretical underpinning of the Framework is that varying external conditions and circumstances will produce different case study results. A large number of cases was therefore included, involving communities that do not usually follow similar courses of health with varying conditions, ethnic, socio-economic, and other differences. The contexts of these cases are likely to differ, so if we arrive at common conclusions across a number of cases with diverse circumstances, we have immeasurably increased the external generalisability of findings (Yin 2014).

In this research, the case is defined as a phenomenon (Carolan, Forbat, and Smith 2016), namely emotional experiences of marginalised communities in different settings. Participants in each case were purposively selected as they had opted to take part in creative, community-based, participatory action research evaluations linked to health and well-being in Scotland from 2013 to 2021.

In Case 1, twenty self-identified Gypsies used music to co-produce a service where they could be supported as they tackled addictive behaviours, stress, and transference of maladaptive coping mechanisms. Detailed findings from Case 1 (de Andrade and Angelova 2020) were used to pilot and test the Framework and problematise evidence and evaluation in asset-based approaches.

In Case 2, 127 secondary school pupils (sixteen to eighteen-year-olds) in fourteen mainstream and three assisted-learning schools in and around areas of multiple deprivation took part in a music and skills programme delivered by industry professionals.

In Case 3, thirty-four community members suffering from, or at risk of, poor mental health engaged with outdoor activities, including environmental art in green spaces. In Case 4, eight members from the Deaf community, four British Sign Language (BSL) interpreters, and seven health-care professionals engaged in a comedy workshop with a famous Deaf comedian exploring mental health issues to inform local community plans and national legislation (BSL [Scotland] Act 2015).

In Case 5, hundreds of community members across three disadvantaged communities engaged with community workers using an asset-based approach to identify neighbourhood assets that create or sustain health and well-being. This approach calls for equal and active participation of community members in initiatives that best suit their needs, desires, and circumstances so multiple methods of engagement were being used, including creative writing, peer-support, gardening, and language groups.

Data across all cases were collected through community-based participatory action research methods, participant observation, creative evaluations using drawings, flip charts, feedback questionnaires from professionals, and reflexive journals.

Each individual case composed a "whole" study and was conducted as a discrete project feeding into the larger research programme. In each case, convergent evidence was sought to draw findings and conclusions. Each case's conclusions was then regarded as data necessitating replication by other individual cases (Yin 2014)

An abductive approach to conceptualisation and theory-building was used combining both deductive and inductive analysis (Dubois and Gadde 2002; Peirce 2014), starting with the application of the Asset-Based Indicator Framework.

Figure 5.1 details stage 1 of the Framework (Process), which was followed by the identification and definition of indicators (emotions and attributes linked to health and well-being) by community members in each case. Thirteen indicators with academic definitions were identified in the literature and served as a template for applications of the co-produced Framework in each case (de Andrade and Angelova 2017). Community members decided if any of these attributes related to them, and defined them accordingly.

This first layer of analysis was followed by an iterative process of reading and coding data under key emergent themes, then critically analysing them using the theory of constructed emotion. Ontologically, these cases present "experiential loose ends that characterise lived lives" of marginalised communities and as such do not present "sanitised measurements" of a single objective reality (Gabb 2009). Implications are expanded in the discussion and conclusion.

The researcher has extensive experience engaging with vulnerable groups. She is also well-versed in using humanities and arts-informed methodologies that necessitate additional ethical deliberation such as management of audio-visual materials to minimise stigma and protect participants. Further ethical

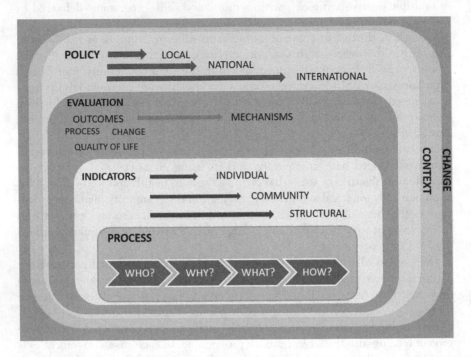

Figure 5.1 The Asset-Based Indicator Framework

Source: copyright belongs to Marisa de Andrade and Nikolina Angelova for the Measuring Humanity project.

considerations are presented elsewhere (de Andrade and Angelova 2020). Ethical approval was granted by the School of Health in Social Science Research Ethics Committee at the University of Edinburgh.

5.1.4 Findings

Limitations of self-reported emotions

Communities across all cases identified emotions (or attributes) that they believe relate to their well-being and circumstances at a community level (see Appendix). This is unsurprising given the universal nature of these attributes and the fact that these measures – with definitions from academic literature – were made available to them at the start of evaluations.

If communities believed that other indicators more accurately reflected their state of being (for example, "autonomy/independence" in Case 1 and "willingness/openness/confidence/sharing" in Cases 2, 3, and 5) (flip charts), they were eager to disclose this. However, there was clear contention within groups when trying to agree on "what should be measured," and dominant voices secured the measure and definition that was finally "accepted," albeit coercively, by the group (field notes). There was also a distinct sense of "gaming" – an awareness that they needed to arrive at a consensus to achieve organisational outcomes (Lowe and Wilson 2017), but these did not necessarily align with community outcomes.

"We move at the speed of trust" was one of the maxims used in Case 5's approach to community engagement, noting that without building trust first, the process of collecting data linked to emotional well-being would lack the integrity needed to carry out authentic, citizen-led community transformation. However, community members questioned how data would be used, and the notion that self-reported measures would lead to improved lived experiences given their circumstances (practitioner field notes).

In Case 3, practitioners said the Warwick-Edinburgh Mental Well-being Scale and another mental health questionnaire were "not ideal" as they were "difficult to use in the field" (video). The overall view was that there was some value in the forms, but they are problematic, so creative data collection methods should be used to evaluate emotional attributes linked to community health. Practitioners further explained how some participants, especially teenagers and vulnerable adults with mental health problems, "don't understand the forms properly" and find putting a number to their emotions difficult. The question "How happy do you feel today on a scale of 1 to 10?" can "change week to week quite dramatically" (video, questionnaires).

Furthermore, filling out forms "is not a simple thing," especially with a community with learning difficulties. For example, a group with learning difficulties was asked to complete evaluation questionnaires assessing changes in emotional well-being at the start of their community intervention, then again at the end. Practitioners explained, "Happiness levels at the end of the group had gone down, because it was the last session. The group enjoyed the last few sessions. They were told there were no more. They said they weren't happy. This is not what they were being asked, but that's what they thought we [practitioners] were asking them" (video).

Practitioners were convinced that the programme improved mental health, but noted that participants' interpretations of questionnaires told a different story. They added that participants were also "unhappy" at that moment as they were being asked to fill in a form rather than take part in the activity they had signed up for (video).

Similarly, in Case 2, questionnaires on the most prevalent indicators – confidence, optimism, social connectedness, and self-determination – produced relatively meaningless data, contradicting what had been observed and expressed by practitioners and other participants. For example, practitioners observed significant changes in confidence in pupils, evident in their increasingly assertive lyric writing, self-expression, and performing to an audience of 500 people.

In evaluation surveys, however, only 60 percent of pupils said their confidence had improved "loads." Similarly, pupils and practitioners spoke optimistically in music sessions about feelings of achievement and how their experience of creating their own tracks, videos, and logos made them feel more optimistic. However, only 37 percent strongly agreed that they "feel more optimistic about the future" after taking part in the intervention (questionnaires, video).

Same emotion, different emotional experience

Once a high-level emotional category was agreed in each case, it became evident that categories meant something different to each group. Happiness, for example, was identified in each community as linked to health and well-being.

In Case 1, it was defined as "sports, music, dance, parties, support, friends, helping people, holidays, achieving your goals, feeling good about your children" (flip charts, video). These conceptualisations of happiness linked to community needs, desires, and gatherings make sense in the Gypsy collectivistic culture, which prioritises the group over each individual. In contrast, happiness was linked to creativity, freedom, and self-expression in Case 2.

In Case 3, happiness was attributed to "the fact that people keep coming through some of the worst weather . . . blizzards and rainstorms" (video). Participants explained how they looked forward to sessions, felt "less stressed" when taking part, and were "unhappy when they miss sessions" (video). While in Case 4, happiness had a bittersweet quality related to how isolated the Deaf community feels and their need to unite and share discontent. Happiness – or relative happiness – was related to the extent to which community members were able to manage and respond to daily challenges in a system that discriminates against them and neglects to understand their lived experiences (video, field notes).

In Case 5, the construct was linked to local connectors and youth raising the profile of community assets through celebration events and videos highlighting positive aspects of their neighbourhoods. Happiness also meant opportunities for community members to voice their views at conversation cafés and listening events (field notes).

It was evident that while groups identified with the same categorised emotion, their unique emotional experiences were closely linked to both individual circumstances and broader cultural and systemic issues.

Subjective emotional experiences, trauma, and the system

Community members were drawn to these creative interventions to focus on positive aspects of life in respective communities, leading to improved health. Once they settled into their groups and began trusting peers and facilitators, however, they started sharing deeply personal and often-troubled experiences relating to harmful or life-threatening events or circumstances with negative impacts on their well-being.

In Case 5, practitioners explained how it "took a lot of digging and persistence to get individuals and organisations to talk about issues that are unproductive to community life" as "most citizens are programmed to exchange polite chat and not discuss anything remotely political." Once community members were "mobilised to talk about issues that are largely going on below the radar of most of the population in [the neighbourhood]," it became apparent that they were experiencing varying degrees of trauma and "find themselves trapped by the issues identified" (practitioner field notes).

Addiction, isolation, and homelessness are examples of systemic issues that emerged through discussions about emotional experiences linked to community health. In the absence of support and access to services, community champions hosted weekly recovery groups to provide social opportunities to share experiences. Practitioners spoke of the "great deal of social skills [needed] to sensitively navigate the relationships that began to emerge with individuals" as they shared distresses in informal community settings by simply "sitting down and making someone a cup of tea, doing the washing-up together at the community lunch, discussing music, reading a poem together, or asking after someone's sick relative." They also spoke of the need to "connect authentically" with traumatised individuals and listen as they shared additional challenges, such as food and fuel poverty, loneliness and isolation, mental ill health, and complex family situations (practitioner field notes).

Similarly, in Case 3, participants on the outdoors programme often used the sessions to reflect on their own difficulties, relying on facilitators for support. For many, the programme was "their only social opportunity." Poverty was also an issue for some participants, who could not attend some sessions as they "didn't have the bus fare or fuel . . . to visit the benefits agency or a food bank" (video).

In Case 1, participants linked racism to poor health outcomes and explained how they hid their identities out of fear of being discriminated against. While in Case 4, a Deaf community member spoke about experiences of not being able to receive psychological support as a BSL interpreter was unavailable. When she began to self-harm, a family member tried to call her psychologist, who was unable to discuss the situation due to data protection. This resulted in a call to emergency services and home visit from two police officers. Upon realising they, too, did not have access to an interpreter, they used the Deaf community member's ten-year-old daughter as a BSL interpreter to explain that her mother needed to go to the hospital and refusing to do so could get her detained. This led to further isolation and emotional distress, and the participant's decision to withdraw from psychological treatment.

Creative interventions for emotion regulation and coping

Music, poetry, environmental art, green space activities, and comedy provided opportunities to downregulate intense emotions and process traumas. In each case, participants and practitioners reflected on how creative media helped them work through difficult emotions and express them constructively. For example, the act of making music in Case 2, or "the expression," was considered by facilitators to be the most accurate form of data or "piece of evidence" as it was not dependent on participants' moods or distractions, such as responding to phone messages when completing surveys. Instead, the process of making music and producing tracks provided "a place where you can expose yourself, where you can let your emotions out." This – described as the "one of the beauties of music" – was described as "hugely positive" by facilitators, even if tracks expressed difficult emotions (video).

All groups in Case 2 wrote and performed original songs. Young participants, who felt inhibited at the start of the sessions and lacked confidence to express emotions in front of peers, opened up as the programme progressed to share feelings of isolation and loneliness through their lyrics: "I'll isolate myself, 'til there's no safety net. . . . Are we the ghost in a crowded room?" (video, track).

According to facilitators, "the level of writing and genuine expression well surpassed our [their] expectations," which was attributed to the "supportive environment and community spirit." Facilitators noticed a marked improvement in participants' communication, confidence, teamwork, and responsibility. In early rehearsals, some participants tended to play "a blame game" by pointing fingers at others who were uncertain of their parts or felt nervous performing in front of others. By encouraging teamwork and an attitude of helping each other with parts they were struggling with, proficient players became mentors to beginners. By final rehearsals, the group dynamic had shifted considerably (practitioner field notes).

In Case 5, the youth wanted to develop documentaries showing how their community supported them and provided a sense of belonging. Community members also used gardening sessions and conversation cafés to learn crafting, singing, and cooking skills while sharing experiences of mental health. Creative writing sessions emerged from a group who used the local food bank and expressed an interest in the medium. Some had begun writing their life story as a way of coming to terms with past traumas; others used poetry to make sense of present circumstances. A published author led locals through creative writing exercises focused on citizens' relationships with the place they were in, both physically and psychologically (practitioner field notes).

Elsewhere in the community, the Buddy Group provided a safe space for children from complex families to meet other children and express themselves creatively through facilitated discussions about an aspect of friendship. This led on to a craft activity linked with that aspect of friendship to allow children dealing with traumatic family bereavements, autism, and siblings with additional support needs to explore what friendship and relationships meant to them (practitioner field notes).

In Case 3, participants took photographs that were used as prompts for personal storytelling during "tea-drinking sessions." A picture of "an empty hammock" – "The Hammock of Happiness" – for example, captured a hammock-building session and was symbolic of the process of connecting and sharing life stories. Environmental art allowed participants to create artefacts and "express themselves" with natural materials. Reflecting on how ancestors, "Forest Guardians," or fellow community members would feel about the art was crucial to the process. Practitioners highlighted the importance of self-expression in whatever form worked for community members, and reflected on how "being creative and coming together opens up this space" to enhance well-being (video, practitioner field notes).

5.1.5 Discussion

As the link between emotions and health is well-established, public health has turned its efforts to understanding, measuring, and promoting emotional well-being alongside prevention and behaviour change. Reasons for this are well-documented: "global affective states – feeling good or bad – contribute to unhealthy behaviours," including smoking, eating, or drinking alcohol excessively (Ferrer et al. 2015).[15]

It follows that changes in emotions are associated with non-communicable health epidemics, such as cancer, cardiovascular and respiratory diseases, chronic respiratory diseases, diabetes, and obesity, so health interventions could benefit from an understanding of the role of emotion in decision-making. Ferrer and colleagues (Ferrer et al. 2015),[16] however, raise an important consideration: "The influence of emotion on interpersonal attribution [seeking others to perceive us positively] may also play a prominent role in health behaviours, particularly when those behaviours are motivated in part by social norms or take place in a social context."

This thinking provides a useful segue into Barrett's (Barrett 2017) theory of constructed emotion, which asserts that while we may all feel the same emotions, we will interpret, experience, and express them differently. Evidence from these neuroscience studies, which include four meta-analyses synthesising hundreds of experiments, highlight the unpredictability and variability of emotions. For me, sadness may feel nourishing; you may experience anger as exhilarating. Consider how happiness had different meanings and qualities in this study's varying contexts and individual circumstances, questioning self-reported measures of emotions. If self-reports are advantageous in that they have good validity and can be easily replicated, they are disadvantageous as fixed-choice questions or Framework prompts lack flexibility and force people to answer in particular ways, thereby lowering validity.

In community contexts, as illustrated in these Cases, there is also evidence of acquiescence bias – reluctantly accepting categorisations without much protest, possibly due to social desirability bias and interpersonal attribution – providing "good, less stigmatising answers" to be viewed favourably by other community members, researchers, practitioners, and policymakers.

According to Barrett (Barrett 2017), emotional experiences and perceptions are linked to pleasant and unpleasant feelings originating from a constant, internal process called interoception. As an essential ingredient of emotion, interoception is our brain's representation of bodily sensations (such heart rate fluctuations) leading to a range of feelings (such as anxiety). Our physical experiences of the same emotion may also differ. In fact, variation is the norm when it comes to physical changes of emotional experiences in different instances, even within an individual, which casts doubt on physiological and observational measurements that claim to be able to read emotions by tracking facial and body movements.

Crucial to the theory of constructed emotion is that whether or not these sensations transform into emotions, they still influence our thoughts, perceptions, and actions:

> *Everything you feel is based on prediction from your knowledge and past experience. . . . You might think that in everyday life, the things you see and hear influence what you feel, but it's mostly the other way around: that what you feel alters your sight and hearing. Interoception in the moment is more influential to perception, and how you act, than the outside world is.*
>
> (Barrett 2017)[17]

This provides a powerful entry point to explore how a person's "inner world" (or subjective reality) collides with "outside-world" systemic issues (for example, the objective reality of inequality). In this study's Cases, community members are clearly affected by traumas, cultural norms, and systemic issues, such as poverty. How they experience emotions (for example, by internalising distress caused by socio-economic inequalities or familial difficulties) or perceive them in others, however, largely depends on what is happening inside their minds – or, according to this theory, how they categorise concepts to make interoceptive sensations meaningful. Contrary to the classical interpretation of concepts, which assumes that categories have rigid boundaries, occurrences of flexible, dynamic, and context-dependent categories are remarkably different from one another.

The implications of findings, through this lens, raise uncomfortable questions for public health interventions, evaluation, and the policies and practices they are informed by reductionist measures of emotions. As Barratt states frankly:

> *Any summary of the population is a statistical fiction that applies to no individual. And most importantly, variation within a species is meaningfully related to the environment in which individuals live.*
>
> (Barrett 2017)[18]

So where do public health interventions, evaluations, and resulting policies go from here?

5.2 Thinking with magical realism

How would these one-dimensional findings reporting on reports of trauma, emotional distress, and poor health change when "plugging in" "enchantment, magic and spirituality" (Laws 2016)?[19] How could an approach that centres on the "more-than-rational"[20] produce more meaningful insights for public health research, policy, and practice?

As I write these words and move further away from a fixed framework and "validated" analytical lens in my field, my feeling as a researcher is that I'm doing something wrong. Something that isn't allowed. Something that doesn't belong here (scientific health research) but belongs over there (creative humanities and arts).

This writing coincides with my work as moderator on a course in clinical psychology that reminds me of the need to treat adolescent mental health problems before they develop into adulthood. This academic literature reinforces the idea that psychosis is very much about people losing touch with reality and feeling or hearing things that aren't "there" and aren't "true." That we should be on the lookout for those, like my Community Members, who have abused drugs or alcohol or experienced trauma (Patel et al. 2014). That we should help them with antipsychotics (despite known side effects) (Tiihonen 2016), with cognitive behaviour therapy (though this is subjective, so we don't really know if it works) (Thomas 2015), or through effective family-based interventions (though family has been the source of trauma for several of the Community Members I've spoken to) (Patel et al. 2014).

I can't ignore that this pathological positioning jars with the human experiences I've encountered in the field. No amount of categorising or "measuring" of emotions got me remotely close to understanding the depths of the trauma and distress that impact poor health. Each deeply personal emotional experience is unique and linked to individual circumstances as well as broader cultural and systemic issues.

I can hear The Community poking at the limitations of the "mainstream evidence base" and being critical of the "pyramids of evidence in which only the tightest clinical trials make top ranks or the traditional division between scientific and magical or sane and mad affairs that organise ordinary discourse" (Laws 2016).[21]

I can feel how their "interpretations of [my] interpretations" take on "significance not for their truth value or inherent meaning, but for the ways in which they disrupt or sustain relations of power and advance knowledge." Community Members "interpret[ting] their situations to both accommodate them and struggle against them to disrupt, contest, and re-signify" (Jackson and Mazzei 2012).[22]

I can imagine them staging an intervention. Inviting me to simply *be with* their experiences of reality.

***

Horizontal rain cuts through the huddle of Community Members, who one by one curl themselves into little balls on the ground, covering themselves with cardboard boxes.

In-Credible doesn't move. She can't quite figure out what's going on.

"If you're wanting to stay dry, you might want to find a box and cover yourself," Sara suggests as she settles into her new home. "What's the problem? You've never been homeless?"

In-Credible grudgingly pulls a punnet over her head, thinking about the times she's found herself between properties, crashing in friends' spare rooms.

"I've been homeless," she says as she meets Sara on drenched concrete. "Listen, I appreciate you going through all this trouble, but I just need to know the truth now so I can go home with the answers we need. What's wrong with you? What's going on in your head? How can we help you?"

Sara smiles. "You want to know the truth? You really want to know what's going on?"

"I wouldn't have come all this way, ignored Professor Ebba . . . risked a discipli-nary hearing at The Institution for not following protocols . . . look, I just need answers now . . ." In-credible shivers, thinking about the consequences of her actions. "Why didn't you follow the Protective Order? Who's Sam, anyway? And what's with Numinous?"

"Okay, you want the truth, so look up." Sara points at the virtual desktop, where a series of colossal emails have appeared.

"What's that?"

"My Downloads. My thoughts, emails, diary entries . . . data. Evidence even. It's all yours."

In-Credible sits up, looks at the scores of documents piling onto the screen.

"When I got back, after breaching my Protective Order, they put me in a glass room on the twenty-seventh floor of the Veritas building. They medicated me to the eyeballs until I levelled out and had enough 'insight' to talk to someone that could help me in a way that made 'sense.' I was stuck there for days, weeks . . . I don't know, maybe months . . . with nothing but my phone, a bed, and a view to the sky."

Sara's inbox appears, filtered to one particular conversation.

"Thankfully, Sam reached out to me. He found me.

In-Credible begins to speed-read.

From: Sam Tambor <sam.tam@veritasinc.com>

Sent: 3 April 15:32:42

To: Sara Aeron<sara.aer@veritasinc.com>

Subject: I found her;-)

[A petite Pine Marten. A Pine Martenette. Almost orange. Lies on a small yellow dinghy floating in the ocean. All around her, there's water everywhere. No land in sight. And it's sunny. A bit like today. So she's wearing her black sunglasses, squinting at the sun. Hands casually clasped behind her head as if she doesn't have a care in the world.]

[WORDS]

In search of truth and destiny, she flees The Futile Forest fast. Surrendering to the journey, she finds total freedom at last.

.

.

.
.
.

I sit back as layer upon layer upon layer of unprocessed thoughts and memories and nightmares and dreams hit me like my emails just did when I opened my laptop.

Are they all just accumulating? Amounting to nothing?

What am I supposed to do with all this untreated information?

My fingers are drawn to the keyboard. The words come out before I can stop them.

.
.

.

From: Sara Aeron<sara.aer@alive.com>
Sent: 6 April 23:28:29
To: Sam Tambor <sam.tam@veritasinc.com>
Subject: RE: I found her;-)

Incredible.

I'll check the Rules to clarify, but think this means you're not just another Community Member but actually The Chosen One. ;-)

As a special treat for your efforts, I've attached a picture of Pine Marten Pat in her spiritual home – The Futile Forest.

[Picture of a statuette of a petite Pine Marten. A Pine Martenette. Almost orange. Lies on a small yellow dinghy floating in the ocean. All around her, there's water everywhere. No land in sight. And it's sunny. A bit like today. So she's wearing her black sunglasses, squinting at the sun. Hands casually clasped behind her head as if she doesn't have a care in the world. She's in her spiritual home – The Futile Forest – surrounded by butterflies and Bodhi trees.]

How's reality treating you?

.
.

.

.

I press Send before I can change my mind.

What have I just done?

A little bit of panic bubbles beneath the surface of my Self. The Self I keep hidden from everyone, including myself.

It's bedtime,

                                   I tell myself.

                                              Time to try to sleep before tomorrow

comes,
                    I tell myself.
                              Tomorrow
is another day,
                    and none of today
                              will matter.
I crawl into bed.

>

>

From: Sam Tambor <sam.tam@veritasinc.com>
Sent: 7 April 11:28:44
To: Sara Aeron<sara.aer@alive.com>
Subject: RE: I found her;-)

I am honoured to be so highly regarded in the Thought Empire, which appears to be a place of infinite wisdom – from metamorphosis to trees of knowledge. I think I need to tap back into the Gateway, though, in order to gain proper passage. ;-)

Needless to say, reality has not been so sublime compared to "our" life in a City in Europe. I keep having random flashbacks, and Behind the Noise has been playing on a constant loop in my mind.

How long did you keep living the magic before reality started to sink back in The Community?

>

>

From: Sara Aeron<sara.aer@alive.com>
Sent: 7 April 23:53
To: Sam Tambor <sam.tam@veritasinc.com>
Subject: RE: I found her;-)

I'm still living the magic. And the flashbacks keep coming thick and fast.

Being back has been as I predicted. I needed the break. I needed to get away. But they didn't want me to get away, Sam. The situation is exactly as I left it. There's still so much truth left to uncover. So much of reality to reveal.

Nothing like the magic we lived. Or whatever that was.

The universe didn't disappoint when I got back to The Community either. There was a random market seller on the high street selling melons. We don't usually get that kind of thing here.

On my way back from the airport, I saw a 4DX banner advert for a new holiday resort in a City in Europe right by the park where we befriended Oracle Man. No word of a lie.

I told the people here all about our experience. I don't think they believe. Convinced I need psychiatric treatment.

So help me out here, Sam. Who are you? Where did you come from? Do we really have a holiday home in a City in Europe? And do you still have access to the Thought Empire?

>

>

From: Sam Tambor <sam.tam@veritasinc.com>
Sent: 8 April 9:44:27
To: Sara Aeron<sara.aer@alive.com>
Subject: RE: I found her;-)
Awesome.
Glad to hear the universe is continuing to serve you in my absence.
Speaking of faraway lands, I present you His Royal Highness, the Oracle Man.
[A man. Crinkled in the face. Dreadlocked in the hair. Impossible to age.]
Psychiatric treatment? Nonsense. I had never met someone so in touch with their inner spiritual Self before meeting you. It's up to us to decide reality from magic. And away we go . . .

I, a young human from a distant land (The State), was cruising the Mediterranean Sea (forbidden territory) in my boat (plane), letting the sea decide where to take me (Pine Marten Pat reference), when suddenly I arrived on the shores of an exotic and unknown land (City in Europe). Upon docking my boat (flight landing), my wandering eyes came across a mysterious human walking along the nearby shores (travelator). Overcome with intrigue, I made haste in approaching this beautiful soul. When I asked for her name and she replied, "Sara" (meaning "pure"), I knew that the fateful currents (missed flight) of the Mediterranean had guided me straight to her. I persuaded Sara to travel farther inland with me along the riverbanks in my boat (now bullet train) by promising her grand tales of adventure and bountiful treats (Truth Bombs), for surely this was the land of such delights. We found refuge at a place of shelter (hotel) perfectly located in the city centre, which quickly became our home away from home . . .

As the years (hours) passed us by, we explored every contour of the local lands, as well as body and mind in a way that transcended reality. We did as the locals did (most popular square in a City in Europe) and befriended the town mystic (Oracle Man), who proved instrumental in guiding us along our journey. Over time, we settled in our holiday home (plot of grass under the Bodhi tree), where Sam and Sara had spent many a days (minutes) basking in the sunlight while gazing in awe at the constantly changing landscape (staring at people) . . .

And life went on as is.
Feel free to edit the above script as you see fit . . .
>
>
From: Sara Aeron<sara.aer@alive.com>
Sent: 9 April 21:24:37
To: Sam Tambor <sam.tam@veritasinc.com>
Subject: RE: I found her;-)
~~Ha ha. You're funny! That's okay, but~~
~~Not bad for a first draft. But a few minor edits . . .~~
I, a mystical human from a spiritual realm few mere mortals travel to (Planet Pine Marten Pat), was chugging wine to drown out reality and staring into the abyss when a vision appeared. I knew at once the human before my very eyes had the power within to secure entry to the Thought Empire.

With an open mind, they were lured by the Gatekeeper. It wasn't long before they tapped into the Gateway (star on a chain around my neck):

[A Seven-Pointed Star. A gift from the spiritual realm to humans to bridge understanding and connection to myself, others, the world, reality, the universe. Each point is a gateway or path of the Higher Self.
Determination
Unconditional love
Awakening
Harmony
Powers of the mind and science
Honesty
Mysticism]

There were, of course, several challenges ahead – this to be expected. There are always obstacles on the path that need to be overcome for true change to happen.

As time moved forward (it never moves back), and Human and Human merged in mind and matter, it became clear that this was no ordinary person, but The Chosen One.

So let's revisit Rule #4: we're scripting this (life).

I've returned to a temporary dwelling (this glass room) with evidence (my memories) from our trip. Everything appears to be the same on the outside (external reality), but everything feels different on the inside (internal reality).

I know that life will never be the same again, but I'm stuck. Stuck in this glass room.

I wish there were some way I could prove what I'm feeling is real. I want to get out of here. I need to get out of here, Sam.

I need some evidence to confirm that you're part of the mortal, human realm and not a spiritual apparition.

Any chance you can help me out?

.

.

.

.

.

Okay. Nothing to do now. Except wait.

Ping.

Ping.

Bzzzzz.

Zing.

The sound of everything but my email alert.

I reach for my phone. Eleven messages from Numinous. Three voicemails.

Pang.

Pang.

Grrro . . .

. . . *wwll.*

The sound of hunger.

I reach for my phone. Open the app they said I should use when I wanted to get my food brought in.

FLASHING BANNER [20 percent off Bodhi tree bonsais!]
MY ACCOUNT [dropdown menu]
ORDER [drinks]
SELECT [1 2 water]
FLASHING BANNER [Summer in a City in Europe!]
CHECKOUT
PAY [amount due: ~~92,099]
ORDER [food]
SELECT [1 Mac and Cheese   1 Steamed Cabbage   1 Jelly]
CHECKOUT
PAY [amount due: ~~153,099]
PAYMENT TYPE [liability card/subsistence allowance]
SCAN [fingerprint/iris]

I turn my phone to silent. Vibrator off.

Okay. Now what.

Ding-dong.

I get the door. A man in a white coat hands me a tray with the goods. Shuts the door behind him.

Pong.

The unmistakable sound of my inbox.

>

>

From: Sam Tambor <sam.tam@veritasinc.com>
To: Sara Aeron<sara.aer@alive.com>
Date: 9 April 22:18:17
Subject: RE: I found her;-)

Spiritual apparition I may just be. I could have sworn you were a mere figment of my imagination until I discovered this gem, which confirmed your existence in the mortal human realm.

A cheesy macaroni falls from my mouth onto the bed. An imaginary hand grabs my heart and squeezes until my left pinky gets pins and needles. Pepper pops in my throat. I'm alternating coughs and wheezes. Tears pour from my tingling eyeballs.

I stare at the photograph Sam's sent me. It's faded a bit. As if scanned from a print that's been stored in a box in someone's attic for decades. It looks like a copy of a snap that's been crumpled into a ball, thrown away, then smoothed out again, in a desperate attempt to get it back to its original form.

I zoom in.

I barely recognise her. But there's no mistaking it. She's definitely me. Caught midlaughter. Guffawing like a buffoon.

I remember the day as if it were today. The prelude to the winter of doom, about a week or so before The Tipping Point. It was almost Christmas, and there should have been so much love in the air. Everywhere you went, you should have smelt cinnamon and roasted chestnuts and pine and log fires and snow.

Clean. Cold. Comforting. Warm.

But something wasn't right. He had cracked one of his rare side-splitting jokes. His gags were usually horrors, but when one of these gems came out between all his cracker jokes, you couldn't contain yourself.

When I finally stopped convulsing, he grabbed me by the waist and spun me 'round and 'round and 'round.

Then he whispered in my ear, "I love you to the moon and back."

Totally impractical, but I believed him. Anything felt possible.

What happened next was impossible to imagine. Impossible to remember.

My hands shake as I drain a cup of water. Stare at my phone some more as if it'll give me all the answers I need.

It all happened so quickly.

Time moves forward; it never moves back.

How? How is this possible?

I remember that moment, but no one was there to take this photo. We were alone in a rented holiday home near a secluded beach. We hadn't seen humans in days. It felt like the end of the world. Apocalyptic. Little did we all know it was just about to be the end of the world – as we knew it. He'd somehow had a premonition about the chaos and hidden us away just as everything began to fall apart. Just as the world split from one into two. Little did I know what would happen next.

How is this possible?

Is Sam trying to tell me something? Is this some sort of cryptic message? A warning?

>

>

>

From: Sara Aeron<sara.aer@alive.com>
To: Sam Tambor <sam.tam@veritasinc.com>
Date: 9 April 22:18:17
Subject: RE: I found her;-)
Sam . . . are you there? Am I in danger? Help me . . . please.[23]

.
.
.
.

I'm lying on the bed, squinting at the midday sun. I've been lying on the bed, squinting at the sun, then my phone, then the sun, then my phone for five days now. Or is it six? Five, I think. Or six. Feels like a decade. Why hasn't Sam replied?

It's a greenhouse in here. Wall-to-wall glass windows, ceiling to floor. No ventilation. Must open a window. Can't open a window – they're sealed shut. Don't have the strength anyway. My right foot has the shakes, and my insides have been scooped out by an invisible ice-cream man, who's left me shivering from the inside out. How's it possible to have hyperthermia in a greenhouse?

Am I dying? Is this what it feels like at the end just before the Grim Reaper takes you away? Just before he sticks his scythe through your soul and drags you to a place of eternal stillness?

I'm on hold. Jupitina stuck me on hold about four hours ago. Or maybe six. Still, I'm holding, staring at the glass cage surrounded by high-rise buildings.

I can't believe they stick us in glass cages. The lot of us. All cooped up in individualised see-through houses so you never feel alone even though you're isolated. Even though you're alone in your isolated, insulated glass cage. We aren't made to be alone, but we are alone.

"No, I don't think you understand . . . I know I'm not being seen for another few days, but . . . listen . . . you're not listening to me . . . stop talking AT me and listen TO me . . . please . . . can you even hear me? Jupitina, I'll say it one last time. I need to speak to Professor Ebba immediately . . . no, it can't wait . . . I need her on the phone . . . I need her on the phone right now . . . what do you mean what's wrong with me? It's none of your business . . . have you ever heard of confidentiality and boundaries and ethics . . . ? Yes, I know you have access to my file . . . I just need to speak to a human. Do you understand that? What am I saying? Am I losing my mind? Of course you don't understand. You're a machine . . . look, I just need some . . . ."

I squint my eyes at the midday sun. Surely not?

Is that an asteroid? The sun hurtling itself towards my window? A burning blob of fire aimed at my face? Is the sun out of control? What the . . .

AAAHHH!

My phone goes flying along with hundreds of pieces of broken glass as someone crashes through my cage and lands on the floor of my room with a roly-poly.

I stare at the spectacle spread across the tiles. He looks familiar. I'm sure I've seen him before.

"Sara, you're okay!"

"Numinous? Is that you?"[24]

He casually flicks shards of glass off his clothes as he unties elasticised rope from his ankles. "It's me."

I look him up and down from head to toe. "Why are you wearing a wetsuit?"

"Protection, Sara. You try flinging yourself through a window without layering."

I look at the door, expecting security to rush in. No one does. "Um. I think you'll find I won't be flinging myself through a window full stop. What are you doing here?"

"Sara, have you lost it completely? It's been six days. You need to get out of here." He's trying to get out of his makeshift superhero outfit without much success.

"Is that two sizes too small for you?" I ask as his wrist refuses to release itself from a vacuum pack.

"Funny. It's the thickest padding I could find." He manages to wriggle out. I notice he isn't wearing any shoes, just modest-sized, waterproof booties made of the same material as his wetsuit.

A backpack's attached to his shoulders. He unzips it to remove a handheld device that he's loaded with footage. "Watch this," he says.

I watch myself leaving Professor Ebba's cube, walking out of my PIG session six days earlier, getting into an e-Charge. Then black.

"And?"

"And that's it."

"Exactly. What's the big deal?"

"What's the big deal, Sara? That's the last memory you have. The last memory I have of you in The Walled Garden."

"The last memory you have of me in The Walled Garden? I hadn't realised you were in charge of my memories."

"Semantics, Sara. You know what I mean. Without The Walled Garden, you're exposed. Vulnerable. With it, you have protection. I've got your back. SANITY's got your back."

I steady myself. Stand up slowly. Amble along to observe the shattered window.

"Sara, don't you get it? You've gone off grid. You're nothing at the moment. Not a thought, not a memory. Are you even an experience?"

"What are you going on about?" I'm picking up pieces of glass and tossing them out my cage, watch them bounce off the boundaried, concrete courtyard below us. I wonder what we must look like from above. Two imprisoned creatures of the system trapped inside a clink of our own making.

"I'm experiencing this, Numinous. How can this moment not be real? Ow!" A sliver slits my thumb open. Blood gushes down the nightshirt I've been wearing for days. "Is that real enough for you?" I flash my wound in his face.

"I'm not saying this isn't real, Sara." He isn't fazed by the outpouring. Grabs a hand towel from the bedside table, tightly wraps the cloth 'round my gash. "It'll stop in a minute." He sits on the edge of the bed. "I'm saying you're suspended in an altered state of reality that doesn't exist. And Sam has something to do with this, Sara. Sam's trouble."

"Sam? What's Sam got to do with this?" My right fist is pumping my left thumb to stop the bleeding.

He reaches for his device. Taps in a password, hits the Play button. Footage of me in an airport, moving on a travelator, smiling at the person beside me.

Flashbacks.

"Hang on a minute. Why are you going through my memory archives?" I feel invaded. Numinous has given himself access to a truth I want to keep hidden. Even from myself.

"Desperate times call for desperate measures, Sara. Don't worry. I don't normally do this – it's against SANITY's ethics protocol. But you were missing. And I could feel it had something to do with Sam."

We both stare at Sam as they glide along the travelator then looks at me while I awkwardly excuse myself to go to the toilet. Sam starts eyeballing the synth.

"Hang on. What's going on here?" I ask.

"Just watch."

The synth shambles to Sam's side. Starts her highly strung exchange.

She hands Sam something small. Something black.

"Your little black pouch! You see. The synth's handing him your little black pouch!" Numinous is pointing at the device, reacting as if the scene's playing out in real time.

"That's it? That's the big reveal?" I wonder when he last got a good night's sleep. I don't think he rests at all. "You do know that's exactly as it happened? I left my little black pouch on the plane and the hyperactive synth, annoying as she is, saved the day by scanning herself into footage of us together on the travelator and came to find us."

"No, Sara. No. That's what Sam told you. That's not what happened at all."

"Really. What do you get from that video that that tells you otherwise? Exactly what kind of evidence do you have access to that I don't?"

He screws his face up the way he always does when he thinks I'm losing the plot. A kind of condescending scrunch-up of his left eye as his lips pucker 'round an imaginary straw.

"Come on, Sara. It's so obvious. Professor Ebba and Sam are in cahoots."

"Okay, now I know you're losing it completely. I know your job is to be paranoid and suspect the worst because, let's face it, This World is screwed and we're all on a one-way ticket to eternal suffering if we don't expose the truth in a matter of days. But honestly, you've to keep it real. You can't see things that aren't there just because you've convinced yourself that they're true. Come on, Numinous. You need to keep it together. Stay focused here."

Why's he refusing to look at me? Why's he staring out the remainder of the window with that glazed look in his eyes? Is he contemplating leaving the same way he came in? Is he going to jump?

"Numinous? Are you there?"

"You don't get it, Sara. You just don't get it. Sam's dangerous. You're losing yourself in some stupid, magical story just before The End and you can't even see it." His words are void of feeling. There's nothing in his tone except automated information.

I've never seen this side of him. Operational oblivion. As if he's lost the ability to sense, to feel, to understand what it is I'm trying to tell him from my perspective. And my viewpoint, right now, is the most important one. I'm the one who knows that Sam is on our side. I'm the one who knows what it felt like to be with them, to experience them, to connect with them, even if just for a few days. I'm the one who's been communicating with them in our liminal space, through our cryptic conversations that only we can decipher. We've got this. Who is Numinous to tell me otherwise?

"You're wrong. I know you're wrong. You're just going to have to trust me on this. You've shown me nothing to convince me otherwise, and until you have concrete evidence to change my mind, you're going to have to believe me when I say that Sam's on our side. We've totally got this."

I see a flicker of something in his eyes. He's a gentle, almost-childlike being. Timid and scared, his eyes are now telling me a different story. One of fear. One of desperation.

"Okay, Sara. If you say so." There's feeling in his words this time. "I hope you know what you're doing here." He blinks to hold back tears. "I just care about you, okay? You're very important to me. I can't bear the thought of anything happening to you."

I wish I had something meaningful to say back, but I have nothing. Emptiness. A void.

"It's okay," I say. I can't detect any emotion in my voice. "Everything's going to be okay."

He puts his device back in his backpack, straps it on, walks to the door, opens it, and lets himself out.

I watch him leave from my bed, wondering why he isn't being dragged out by security. Wondering why he didn't just come in through the door, given that he works in the building.

***

Notes

1 Page 961.
2 Page 79.
3 Page 101.
4 "Plugging in" is a phrase on page 4 of Deleuze and Guattari's (1987) *A Thousand Plateaus* to bring to life the image of one "literary machine" needing to be plugged into another for it to work. Jackson and Mazzei (2011) use it to make sense of the numerous co-authored "literary machines" – data, conversations, interviews, theories, peer reviews, etc. – that depend on a "plugging in of ideas, fragments, theory, selves, sensations" as "processes" instead of "concepts" (page 2).

5 Page 6.

6 The following is the Behind the Noise soundtrack to this scene: Listen to "You're Welcome" by Attention Seekers (King's Park Secondary School) by Behind the Noise in Sessions 2018/19 playlist online for free on SoundCloud. https://soundcloud.com/behindthenoise/youre-welcome-by-attention-seekers

7 Direct quotes are lyrics from "You're Welcome" by Attention Seekers, as earlier.

8 John Smith is one of the UK's most famous Deaf comedians. He led the workshops in the Asset-Based Indicator Framework application *Measuring Humanity with the Deaf Community through Comedy* to engage the community on awareness of barriers to mental health services. In this tale of magical realism, he's the inspiration for Mark Rodger.

9 This wording is taken from the publisher's proposal guidelines.

10 Page 21.

11 Pages 6–7.

12 Page vii.

13 Pages 3, 283.

14 Full report on community-centred approaches for health and well-being: (Public Health England 2015).

15 Page 3.

16 Page 10.

17 Pages 78–79.

18 Page 94.

19 Page 3.

20 Page 4.

21 Page 59.

22 Ibid.

23 Arva (2008) reminds me that "as a process of the traumatic imagination, magical realist writing keeps alive the illusion and the mystery inherent in phenomenal knowledge, particularly when the object of that knowledge is death or pain" (page 74).

24 Citing the prolific psychiatrist and psychoanalyst Carl Jung, the Religious Studies scholar Leon Schlamm states, "Numinous experiences, identified by Jung with experiences of the unconscious . . . possess a 'deeply stirring emotional effect' . . . 'thrilling power' . . . *mana* (psychic power) equated with holiness, healing or destructive qualities . . . and are therefore unusually persuasive from the psychological point of view. . . . They are independent of conscious volition, transporting 'the subject into the state of rapture, which is a state of will-less surrender.' . . . For this reason, they are 'difficult to handle intellectually, since our affectivity is involved. . . . Absolute objectivity is more rarely achieved here than anywhere else'" (Schlamm 2007) (page 2).

Reference List

Abma, Tineke A., and Robert E. Stake. 2014. "Science of the Particular: An Advocacy of Naturalistic Case Study in Health Research." *Qualitative Health Research* 24 (8): 1150–61. https://doi.org/10.1177/1049732314543196.

Arva, Eugene L. 2008. "Writing the Vanishing Real: Hyperreality and Magical Realism." *JNT-Journal of Narrative Theory* 38 (1): 60–85. https://doi.org/10.1353/JNT.0.0002.

Barrett, Lisa. 2016. "Navigating the Science of Emotion." *Emotion Measurement* (January): 31–63. https://doi.org/10.1016/B978-0-08-100508-8.00002-3.

———. 2017. *How Emotions Are Made: The Secret Life of the Brain.* Houghton Mifflin Harcourt. https://psycnet.apa.org/record/2017-26294-000.

Bonetti, Debbie, Martin Eccles, Marie Johnston, Nick Steen, Jeremy Grimshaw, Rachel Baker, Anne Walker, and Nigel Pitts. 2005. "Guiding the Design and Selection of Interventions to Influence the Implementation of Evidence-Based Practice: An

Experimental Simulation of a Complex Intervention Trial." *Social Science and Medicine* 60 (9): 2135–47. www.academia.edu/18908046/Guiding_the_design_and_selection_ of_interventions_to_influence_the_implementation_of_evidence_based_practice_an_ experimental_simulation_of_a_complex_intervention_trial.

Butler, Judith. 2001. *Giving an Account of Oneself. Diacritics*. Vol. 31. The Johns Hopkins University Press. www.jstor.org/stable/1566427.

Carolan, Clare M., Liz Forbat, and Annetta Smith. 2016. "Developing the DESCARTE Model: The Design of Case Study Research in Health Care." *Qualitative Health Research* 26 (5): 626–39. https://doi.org/10.1177/1049732315602488.

Ciuk, David, Allison K. Troy, and Markera C. Jones. 2015. "Measuring Emotion: Self-Reports vs. Physiological Indicators." *SSRN Electronic Journal* (April). https://doi.org/10.2139/SSRN.2595359.

Craig, Peter. 2006. "Developing and Evaluating Complex Interventions." www.mrc.ac.uk/complexinterventionsguidance.

de Andrade, Marisa, and Nikolina Angelova. 2017. "An Asset-Based Indicator Framework: Using Co-Production, Co-Design and Innovative Methods to Engage with BME Groups." In *Glasgow Health and Social Care Partnership*, edited by G. Balint, B. Antala, C. Carty, J-M. A. Mabieme, I. B. Amar, and A. Kaplanova. https://doi.org/10.2/JQUERY.MIN.JS.

de Andrade, Marisa, and Nikolina Angelova. 2020. "Evaluating and Evidencing Asset-Based Approaches and Co-Production in Health Inequalities: Measuring the Unmeasurable?" *Critical Public Health* 30 (2): 232–44. https://doi.org/10.1080/09581596.2018.1 541229/SUPPL_FILE/CCPH_A_1541229_SM0659.PDF

de Andrade, Marisa De, Rosie Stenhouse, and Jonathan Wyatt. 2020. "Some Openings, Possibilities, and Constraints of Creative-Relational InquiryIntroduction to the Special Issue." *Departures in Critical Qualitative Research* 9 (2): 1–15. https://doi.org/10.1525/DCQR.2020.9.2.1.

Deleuze, Gilles, and Félix Guattari. 1987. *"A Thousand Plateaus": Capitalism & Schizophrenia*. Translated by Brian Massumi, 4. Minneapolis, MN: University of Minnesota Press.

Dubois, Anna, and Lars Erik Gadde. 2002. "Systematic Combining: An Abductive Approach to Case Research." *Journal of Business Research* 55 (7): 553–60. https://doi.org/10.1016/S0148-2963(00)00195-8.

Ellison, George T. H. 2010. "'Population Profiling' and Public Health Risk: When and How Should We Use Race/Ethnicity?" 15 (1): 65–74. https://doi.org/10.1080/09581590500048416.

Ferrer, Rebecca A., William Klein, Jennifer Lerner, Valerie Reyna, and Dacher Keltner. 2015. "Emotions and Health Decision Making." *Behavioral Economics and Public Health* (November): 101–32. https://doi.org/10.1093/MED/9780199398331.003.0004.

Ferrer, Rebecca A., and Wendy Berry Mendes. 2018. "Emotion, Health Decision Making, and Health Behaviour." *Psychology & Health* 33 (1): 1–16. https://doi.org/10.1080/088 70446.2017.1385787.

Gabb, Jacqui. 2009. "Researching Family Relationships: A Qualitative Mixed Methods Approach." *Methodological Innovations* 4 (2): 37–52. https://doi.org/10.1177/205979910900400204.

Gale, Ken. 2018. *Madness as Methodology: Bringing Concepts to Life in Contemporary Theorising and Inquiry*. New York: Routledge.

Greenhalgh, Trisha, and Chrysanthi Papoutsi. 2018. "Studying Complexity in Health Services Research: Desperately Seeking an Overdue Paradigm Shift." *BMC Medicine* 16 (1): 1–6. https://doi.org/10.1186/S12916-018-1089-4/TABLES/1.

The Health Foundation. 2010. *Complex Adaptive Systems.*

Hekman, Susan. 2010. *The Material of Knowledge: Feminist Disclosures.* Bloomington: Indiana University Press. https://muse.jhu.edu/book/316.

Jackson, Alecia Y., and Lisa A. Mazzei. 2011. *Thinking with Theory in Qualitative Research: Viewing Data Across Multiple Perspectives. The Qualitative Report.* Vol. 20. New York: Routledge.

———. 2013. "Plugging One Text Into Another: Thinking With Theory in Qualitative Research." 19 (4): 261–71. https://doi.org/10.1177/1077800412471510.

Kobau, Rosemarie, Martin E. P. Seligman, Christopher Peterson, Ed Diener, Matthew M. Zack, Daniel Chapman, and William Thompson. 2011. "Mental Health Promotion in Public Health: Perspectives and Strategies From Positive Psychology." *American Journal of Public Health* 101 (8): e1. https://doi.org/10.2105/AJPH.2010.300083.

Laws, Jennifer. 2016. "Magic at the Margins: Towards a Magical Realist Human Geography." *Cultural Geographies* 24 (1): 3–19. https://doi.org/10.1177/1474474016647367.

Loeffler, Elke, Gerry Power, Tony Bovaird, and Frankie Hine-Hughes. 2013. *Co-Production of Health and Wellbeing in Scotland.* Birmingham: Governance International.

Lowe, Toby, and Rob Wilson. 2017. "Playing the Game of Outcomes-Based Performance Management. Is Gamesmanship Inevitable? Evidence from Theory and Practice." *Social Policy & Administration* 51 (7): 981–1001. https://doi.org/10.1111/SPOL.12205.

National Institute for Health and Care Excellence. 2012. "Social and Emotional Wellbeing: Early Years." *Public Health Guideline [PH40].* www.nice.org.uk/guidance/ph40/chapter/2-Public-health-need-and-practice.

Patel, Krishna R., Jessica Cherian, Kunj Gohil, and Dylan Atkinson. 2014. "Schizophrenia: Overview and Treatment Options." *Pharmacy and Therapeutics* 39 (9): 638. /pmc/articles/PMC4159061/.

Peirce, Charles Sanders. 2014. *Illustrations of the Logic of Science.* Edited by Cornelis de Waal. Chicago: Open Court.

Peters, B. Guy. 2017. "What Is so Wicked about Wicked Problems? A Conceptual Analysis and a Research Program." *Policy and Society* 36 (3): 385–96. https://doi.org/10.1080/14494035.2017.1361633.

Plsek, P. E., and T. Wilson. 2001. "Complexity, Leadership, and Management in Healthcare Organisations." *BMJ* 323 (7315): 746–49. https://doi.org/10.1136/BMJ.323.7315.746.

Public Health England. 2015. *A Guide to Community-Centred Approaches for Health and Wellbeing Full Report.* London: Public Health England.

Richardson, Laurel, and Elizabeth St Pierre. 2005. "Writing: A Method of Inquiry." In *The Sage Handbook of Qualitative Research.* Sage Publications Ltf. https://psycnet.apa.org/record/2005-07735-038.

Schlamm, Leon. 2007. "C. G. Jung and Numinous Experience: Between the Known and the Unknown." *European Journal of Psychotherapy and Counselling* 9 (4): 403–414.

Shavers, Vickie. 2007. "Measurement of Socioeconomic Status in Health Disparities Research." *National Medical Association.* https://doi.org/10.1016/S0033-3549(04)50073-0.

Thomas, Neil. 2015. "What's Really Wrong with Cognitive Behavioral Therapy for Psychosis?" *Frontiers in Psychology* 6 (MAR): 323. https://doi.org/10.3389/FPSYG.2015.00323.

Tiihonen, Jari. 2016. "Real-world Effectiveness of Antipsychotics." *Acta Psychiatrica Scandinavica* 134 (5): 371. https://doi.org/10.1111/ACPS.12641.

Yin, Robert. 2014. *Case Study Research: Design and Methods.* Los Angeles, CA: Sage Publications.

6 Convergence – accepting our differences

INTERLUDE – INTEGRATING MULTIPLE SELVES AND INCLUDING MULTIPLE REALITIES IN PUBLIC HEALTH

Will we ever know what happened to Sara with that mystery man on the eve of The Tipping Point, a memory so traumatic it's been blocked out of her consciousness? If Sara doesn't have access to it, if the experience has been pushed away and out of herself, how will we ever have access to her trauma?[1]

How will we ever have access to any of the traumas and experiences of the other Community Members who gather in The Futile Forest and other realms to experience reality and the divine in different ways – as a healing journey or life path – connected to what it truly means to be human?

Will we ever know the truth about The Institution and Veritas Inc. and whether Sam or Numinous were really on Sara's side? Whether they were real or unreal? Whether Sara was in a mental health unit? Psychiatric hospital? Or whether she was experiencing these thoughts at home or on the streets? Was she suffering? Trapped in her own mind? Or was this a liberating, unifying experience for her?[2]

Maybe Sam and Sara together were Sam-Sara, or Samsara – the endless cycle of birth, death, and rebirth in Buddhism – the opposite of Nirvana, which is freedom from suffering and the cycle of rebirth?

Much like the end of Samsara, maybe the end of Sara's endless cycle of suffering from "mental health illnesses" will come from ending the pattern of running away from the pain and throwing herself at a broken system?

What about the other Community Members? Are they all struggling with their mental health? Have they been pummelled by the pathology and politics of madness? Are they lost in their minds? Stuck in a complex web of darkness where they've found bureaucracy, box-ticking, legalities, waiting lists, abuse, addiction, confusion, court orders, confidentiality breaches, organisations covering their own backs and tracks – a system that many of them believe is acting against them in their moment of need?

A system that just doesn't understand them. A system that they believe is messed up. More messed up than they are. A system that they believe wants to measure, capture, and evidence their madness to make it more treatable. To

DOI: 10.4324/9781003196488-6

make it more contained. To make it more manageable. To shame it, inadvertently perhaps. To numb and restrain whatever state of mental disturbance was causing trouble to themselves and to others. To family members, spouses, partners. To colleagues, companies, institutions. To our neighbourhoods, countries, developed and underdeveloped nations. Within homes, at the borders, across borders.

Contradictions and booby traps with every episode.

Help – while sometimes well-intentioned – evoking a sense of helplessness.

There's a mounting body of research that recognises the importance of involving people on the margins and/or those with mental ill health in the "reframing of their own recovery narratives," but "those removed from 'normal' society are generally deemed less capable of independent, coherent thinking" (Fixsen 2021).[3]

As such, the narratives presented in this book may be deemed to be too mind-boggling, interesting – insightful at best – but in no way worthy of inclusion in a public health database to lead to changes in policies and practices.

This is a profound limitation.

Drawing on Jennifer Laws "manifesto for a magically informed method," which she aimed at human geographers, the eloquent invitation for public health is to:

> *Open up scholarly research to include more magic. . . . [by] committing to research methods and cultures of writing that are capable of responding to magic – in which spaces for response and observation are open-ended and unstructured, or in which magic, wonder and the transcendental of everyday interactions form the backbone of question-setting and analysis. . . . [We need to] reject the teaching of uncritical hierarchies of evidence that dismiss unusual, inexplicable and magical happenings . . . be aware and unafraid of what is sometimes strange and unsettling about the mad and magical worlds of people living with enduring psychological distress. Embrace ethics of research in which giving voice to people with mental health difficulties is not conditional upon their conformity to accepted recovery narratives, or in which stories can only be permissible evidence if experiences of magic are retold to match researchers', policymakers' or service providers' own explanations of what they are doing.*
>
> (Laws 2016)[4]

Public health can do so much more with its statistics and qualitative or creative methods, usually positioned as community engagement or participatory action research (PAR). These approaches only scratch the surface of the possibilities that post-qualitative, arts-informed methodologies and theories can bring to the discipline.

There is much to be gained from invigorating conventional approaches to public health by situating ourselves in alternative – sometimes metaphysical – realities where knowledge, evidence, data collection, and analysis take on new meanings for "participants" and researchers. So that "participants" become researchers.

In these realms, commonly understood and experienced emotions take on different meanings for different individuals, even within the same community.

Definitions are closely linked to significant and sometimes traumatic life events and subjectively described – sometimes magically – through personal experiences though are inextricably linked to wider societal and structural issues, such as racism, discrimination, abuse, addiction, and unemployment.

In these realms, it is impossible to instigate a public health intervention, evaluation, and resulting policy linking population health to emotional well-being that can be adequately replicated, and there is no objective way of knowing if someone is in a particular emotional state (Barrett et al. 2019). If emotions are conceptualised, understood, experienced, and expressed differently by different communities – with variances within community groups, too, depending on an individual's makeup and circumstances – then the design, delivery, and evaluation of population-level interventions reliant on this categorised data needs to be reconsidered or could be misleading and ineffective.

By persisting with a standard narrative framework that insists on principles grounded in reductionism that obscure meaningful variations within categories of emotions, we miss out on opportunities to understand narratives behind emotions. We also inadvertently bury relationships between measures that need to be inductively revealed within an individual in varying contexts. Rather than viewing the measurement of emotion through traditional conceptualisations, this invites radical thinking with regards to "measuring" human experience and perception (Barrett 2017).

In these realms, it is very difficult – if not impossible – to objectively put the experience of a feeling or emotion into words. To "validate the feels." There is a difference between how you feel and how others feel about you. Others' observations and recordings during the evidence gathering process may be an inaccurate reflection of the tone or essence of your emotional experience.

If words fall short of articulating emotions and the quality of your emotions comes from sensations in your body, then researchers, practitioners, and policymakers seeking to reduce health inequalities need to incorporate more than purely written forms of data into the evidence-base. Public health's overreliance on text rather than embodied creative-relational methodologies may provide some explanation for repeated failed attempts at understanding what it means to be healthy, what it means to be well, what it means to be human.

We also need to think beyond reductionist box-ticking when assessing rigour. There are different types of knowing (Eisner 2008), and public health needs alternative humanities and arts-informed knowledge to complement and interrogate – or be in conversation with – scientific datasets. This requires science to go beyond replicating experiments to lock down a novel facet of reality, to accepting that the human experience offers a prism of realities that can be creatively navigated to produce new meanings.

As Rachel Horst reflects in her "experimental writing inquiry into future imaginaries":

> Bruner (1991)[5] *suggests that, "narrative organizes the structure of human experience". In the same way that art is an imitation of life, according to Bruner, life becomes an imitation of art. Our plans, dreams, speculations, hopes, fears, and*

ruminations are steeped in narrative futures that connect the present moment to an imagined tomorrow and guide our actions in time with reason and purpose. Our stories have persuasive impact upon the creation of reality and are, therefore, powerful and performative tools for effecting positive change.

Sara's story – as an underexplored counter-narrative in public health research, policy, and practice – may be more liberating for her than the label of "victim of mental illness."

Sam and Sara's magical journey in their minds – trying to make sense of what is real and what is unreal in their internal-external environments – may help us untangle the pathology and inner experience of "mental illness," along with the elation that comes with it when accepted and understood. "Recovery" through this lens is more about self-discovery, healing, and creativity than recuperation.

In essence, the knowing is endless and happens in safe, creative, nourishing relationships.

***

In-Credible peels a wilted cardboard box from her shoulders. In the horizon, she sees a slither of light. Pale blue with a spark of orange and hint of pink, so fierce and intense that for a moment she becomes the sunset. She moves her knotted neck from left to right, left to right – a roll from side to side – weaves her fingers together, then stretches her back like a cat-cow. It's quiet. Deathly quiet.

Using her hands to pin her to the ground, she anchors her left foot then right and rises to standing, one vertebrate at a time, looks around her. Not a soul in sight.

She's in a parking lot at the base of the Beguile Buildings. Her e-Charge is the only vehicle around. There's a notepad and pen at her feet. She bends down to pick it up, recognises her handwriting.

Get inside your data – get Behind the Noise

* Don't think of the "representation" of the research data through "art/ story" – think of the "process of art/story" as being both the data and the research.[6]

* "Data and theory and method . . . never stand alone, isolated and elevated; rather, they keep things on the move, keep things becoming . . . . There is radical possibility in the unfinalized."[7]

So what does all this mean?

* Science can only take us so far in understanding what's going on in the mind of another, what's happening under the skin of another. It can't get in touch with the essence of what makes us feel alive, of what makes us

distressed, triggered, or traumatised. It doesn't have access to our conscious or unconscious thoughts and behaviours.

* Science can't conclusively cognise our values, experiences, and perspectives that are all radically different.

* Maybe our biggest societal win would be to not necessarily make (mental) health problems converge but to acknowledge and explore their existence – their differences, vulnerabilities, and strengths.

*** I feel like I'm touching something that I've never come close to before. This research is so freeing . . . I feel like I'm tumbling into truth like butterflies falling over each . . . ***

In-Credible smiles at her scribbles. Her eyelids feel heavy, her body achy.

She slowly makes her way towards her e-Charge, programmes it to go straight to The Institution. She's exhausted but also invigorated. She has some work to do.

As she sets off in autopilot, her eyes close for a brief moment. It's silent. In her mind, she sees a garden. *I'll call it The Silent Garden*, she thinks as a smile spreads across her lips. It's hovering in the clouds, perched near the stars. A circular green space of epic proportions exposed to the elements.

A helicopter pilot could make out its perfect symmetry from above. Twelve spokes on a wheel, each segment a perfect slice of nature. In the middle, a big Bodhi tree that sheds leaves like a snake sheds skins but never dies. Just constant renewal as long as there is enough water in its roots.

She breathes in the early morning. The air has the smell of starting over. And wet wild mushrooms. She spots one looking like a little palm tree with a sombrero instead of leaves. Another shaped like an oversized golf tee.

There's a great oak still soaking up last night's downpour. A single swallow manifests a fine shower as it flies from branch to twig then takes off like a shuttlecock to join a second swallow in the sky. Together they turn to salmon swimming upstream in unison. In her mind, she blinks several times to bring her eyes back to the reality of the present moment. *Those are birds, In-Credible. Birds. Not fish. Birds, not fish.*

She focuses her attention on a path a woodchuck's carved, kicks small bits of timber as she strolls, then stops to watch a spider doing bondage with a fly in the silkiest of ropes, right beside a bush of purple pincushions scratching the belly of a bee. Thistles. Her favourite. She loves how their lavender shade makes them appear to be gentle even though they're spiky by nature. Hardened edges to protect a softness hidden inside. She picks burnt-orange and white petals from a flower with a mane, its lion face a pursed green tomato.

A butterfly lands on the grass; its furry velvet royal-blue eyes stare her out. *The Secret Garden*, she thinks. *It's watching me.* If it isn't the insects, it's the cameras. Or trees with their wooden eyeballs carved into trunks. The ones on the two rows of eight symmetrically aligned Cigarette Trees are particularly demonic, she thinks. Red rings 'round black pupils etched into thin white bark covered in layers of wood-chipped wallpaper. As you peel off layer upon layer, the one underneath becomes yellower. More nicotine-stained. And little roll-ups like the ones you used to be able to fill with tobacco fall to the earth.

A bumble bee buzzes past her ear, settling in a flower masquerading as a gramophone. She turns right into the forest leading to a Bodhi tree, where she spreads herself across the bench beneath it, stomach to the heavens. The sun squints through leaves like a kaleidoscope. A single white feather floats towards her face as the winds speak over each other.

Yes, she thinks as her phone starts ringing, *I've taken my first step on the path, and there is no going back.*

She clears her throat, opens her eyes. "Hello, Professor Ebba . . . yes, I've got what I came here for. I'm on my way back."

As she hangs up, In-Credible looks through the windscreen on her way out of Beguile. That's when she sees her for the first time, leaning against a broken bus shelter, her pointy shoulder blades piercing the shattered glass that's more disco ball than protective barrier. She's moving to what appears to be trance music that only she could hear, her fragile hips occasionally meeting her flicking fingers. She has no coat to speak of except for a flimsy purple scarf draped ceremoniously at her elbows.

She's about a meter in front of In-Credible, who scans her face for signs of a breakdown. Her edges look surprisingly soft, as if she's dissolving into the grey of the heavens around her. Those black-olive eyes. So alert, attentive, alive.

She looks like Sara. A party girl. Hard to please. Easy on the eye. In-Credible finds herself drawn to her like a moth to a flame, sensing she's about to get burnt, unable to stop some indescribable force. She feels so familiar. It's as if they've met before.

In-Credible feels energised. Conflicted. Her thinking deconstructed. The story she's created about her experience in this Impoverished Community is changing again, she realises. It's already being rewritten, her own narrative overwhelmed and revised with it in this very moment.

Sara looks up just as the e-Charge drives past the bus stop. For a moment, their eyes meet. They're locked into some truth. There's an openness and acceptance.

In-Credible tries to think of a word to capture this moment. There is only one. Magical.

***

Notes

1 As Arva (2008) puts it, "the felt reality recreated by the magical realist image" is an "attempt to reconstruct violent events." It is '"registered' belatedly by characters, narrators, and readers because the 'pressure' of the initial event blocked its complete registration and further narrativization" (page 61).

2 The best I can do here is to create Sara's story as she told it to me as we related, creatively. As we tried to voice the trauma in a safe, creative-relational way. As we co-(re) constructed her reality through magical realism.

3 Page 8.

4 Page 15.
5 Page 5.
6 Horst 2021, page 138.
7 Jackson and Mazzei 2013, page 270.

Reference List

Arva, Eugene L. 2008. "Writing the Vanishing Real: Hyperreality and Magical Realism." *JNT-Journal of Narrative Theory* 38 (1): 60–85. https://doi.org/10.1353/JNT.0.0002.

Barrett, Lisa. 2017. "The Theory of Constructed Emotion: An Active Inference Account of Interoception and Categorization." *Social Cognitive and Affective Neuroscience* 12 (1): 1–23. https://doi.org/10.1093/SCAN/NSW154.

Barrett, Lisa, Ralph Adolphs, Stacy Marsella, Aleix M. Martinez, and Seth D. Pollak. 2019. "Emotional Expressions Reconsidered: Challenges to Inferring Emotion From Human Facial Movements." *Psychological Science in Public Interest* 20 (1): 1–68. https://doi.org/10.1177/1529100619832930.

Bruner, Jerome. 1991. *The Narrative Construction of Reality. Critical Inquiry.* 1st ed. Vol. 18. University of Chicago Press. www.jstor.org/stable/1343711.

Eisner, Elliot. 2008. "Art and Knowledge." In *Handbook of the Arts in Qualitative Research: Perspectives, Methodologies, Examples, and Issues.* Los Angeles: Sage Publications.

Fixsen, Alison. 2021. "'Communitas in Crisis': An Autoethnography of Psychosis Under Lockdown." *Qualitative Health Research* 31 (12): 2340–50. https://doi.org/10.1177/10497323211025247.

Horst, Rachel. 2021. "Narrative Futuring: An Experimental Writing Inquiry Into the Future Imaginaries." *Art/Research International* 6 (1). https://journals.library.ualberta.ca/ari/index.php/ari/article/view/29554/22016.

Jackson, Alecia Y., and Lisa A. Mazzei. 2013. "Plugging One Text Into Another: Thinking with Theory in Qualitative Research." 19 (4): 261–71. https://doi.org/10.1177/1077800412471510.

Laws, Jennifer. 2016. "Magic at the Margins: Towards a Magical Realist Human Geography." *Cultural Geographies* 24 (1): 3–19. https://doi.org/10.1177/1474474016647367.

Public Health, Humanities and Magical Realism: A Creative-Relational Approach to Researching Human Experience

Marisa de Andrade

Table A.1 Summary of fieldwork and means of data collection for selected Measuring Humanity projects

	Who? Definition of Community	Why? Reason for intervention/ evaluation and why implemented at this time	What? Description of intervention/ evaluation	How? Means of data collection	When? Timing of intervention/ evaluation
Case 1 (Roma)	The "Roma" Community, self-identified Gypsies (n=20)	Develop and implement co-produced methodological evaluation framework to measure impacts of creative community engagement on health and inequalities	Six-month ethnography with community members Two seven-hour community-based participatory action research workshops with Gypsies (n=9) and professional stakeholders (n=41) Seven-hour community-based participatory action research singing workshop with Gypsies (n=20)	Music-making and singing Data gathered through video, creative evaluations using drawings, flip charts, feedback questionnaires from professionals, reflexive journal	May 2013– December 2017
Case 2 (schools)	127 secondary school pupils (aged 16–18) in fourteen mainstream and three assisted-learning schools in and around areas of multiple deprivation	Inspire, encourage, and support young people who have an interest in music and careers in the creative sector	Delivered by industry professionals via a series of workshops, rehearsal days, recording sessions, industry panels, and live events where pupils perform and assist in promoting and delivering shows Supervised activities totalling forty-four hours for each group	Music-making (original songs), producing tracks and videos, logo design, feedback questionnaires, interviews, participant observation	October 2018– May 2019

Case 3 (Green Spaces)	Those at risk of mental ill health. Three pilot groups: (i) Neighbourhood networks (n=11, aged 18–54). Participants' health conditions: Sensory – difficulty with sight and/or hearing. Developmental disability – difficulty with language, learning, and/or independent living. Neurological disorders – muscle weakness, seizures, and/or poor coordination. (ii) High school group (n=13, under 16). One participant with a learning difficulty. One wheelchair user. (iii) Open group (n=10, variable as drop-in)	Use the outdoor environment and connect with nature to improve health and well-being. Support and enhance individual and community assets	Variety of session outlines, lengths, and locations trialled, mostly two to three hours outdoors in a natural, green environment. Groups 1 and 2 led by two staff members of staff, group 3 mostly led by one staff member	Observational data – contemporaneous notes taken by project and support staff, semistructured interviews - with project staff and referral partners, focus groups – with participants (at project start and end) of the project, questionnaires from participants (at start and end) capturing measurements of well-being, physical activity levels, and use of local green spaces, and Warwick-Edinburgh Mental Well-being Scale, videos, environmental art	April 2016 and February 2017 (pilot evaluation) going open groups

(*Continued*)

Table A.1 (Continued)

	Who? Definition of Community	Why? Reason for intervention/ evaluation and why implemented at this time	What? Description of intervention/ evaluation	How? Means of data collection	When? Timing of intervention/ evaluation
Case 4 (Deaf Community)	Deaf community (n=8) interested in exploring mental health	Break down barriers and co-produce appropriate services with the Deaf Community and mental health professionals Shape local action plans and legislation particularly in relation to the British Sign Language (BSL) Act Establish unmet needs of BSL users in relation to mental health; improve Deaf people's knowledge of mental health services; establish Best Practice in mental health services/prevention for BSL Explore value of people's stories and experiences expressed through the medium of comedy	Members of the Deaf community (n=8), BSL interpreters (N=4), health-care professionals (N=7) engaged in a four-hour comedy workshop facilitated by a famous Deaf comedian and researcher, evening comedy performance	Comedy and improvisational exercises, interviews, feedback questionnaires, videos	May 2018

| Case 5 | Community members from four Scottish neighbourhoods with multiple inequalities (ongoing) | Apply asset-based community development techniques with citizen-led groups
Build relationships with community leaders of local organisations
Create opportunities for target groups – workless households; individuals facing homelessness or housing challenges; other local disadvantaged groups | Embed community development workers in informal social fabric of areas, hold conversations/creative community engagements informed by community needs and desires | Focus groups, questionnaires, semistructured interviews in locations where hard-to-reach individuals may engage (e.g., food banks, conversation cafés, writing and support groups, gardening and buddy groups, craft-making and language classes, other citizen-led creative community engagements | Phase 1: April 2018–October 2018
Phase 2: 2013–2021 |

Index

Note: Page numbers in italics indicate a figure on the corresponding page. Page numbers followed by 'n' indicate a note.

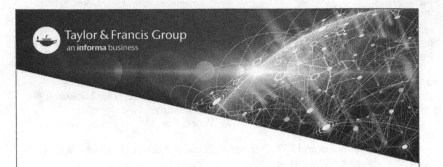

Printed in the United States
by Baker & Taylor Publisher Services

Printed in the United States
by Baker & Taylor Publisher Services